Frontiers in Ophthalmology and Ocular Imaging

Edited by Alireza Ziaei

Published in London, United Kingdom

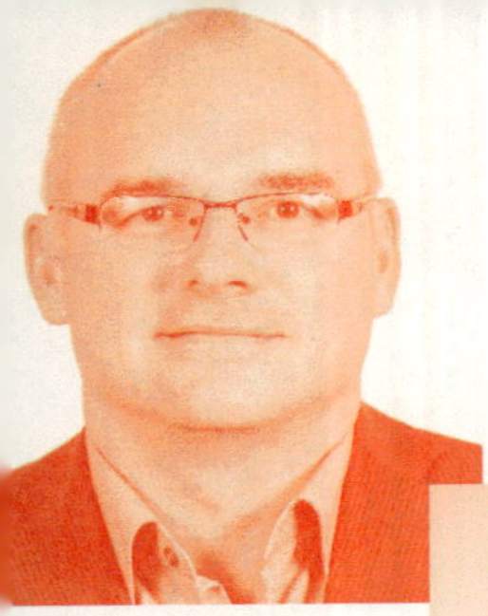
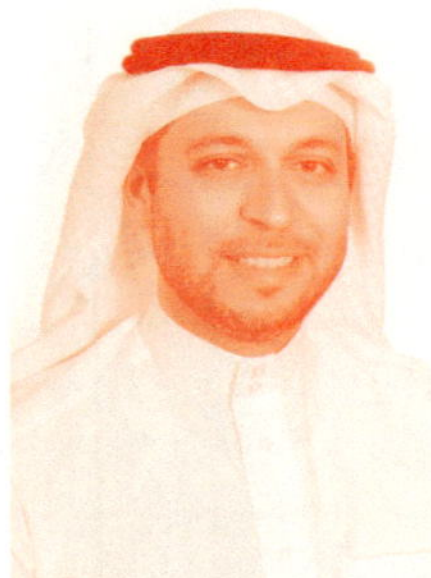
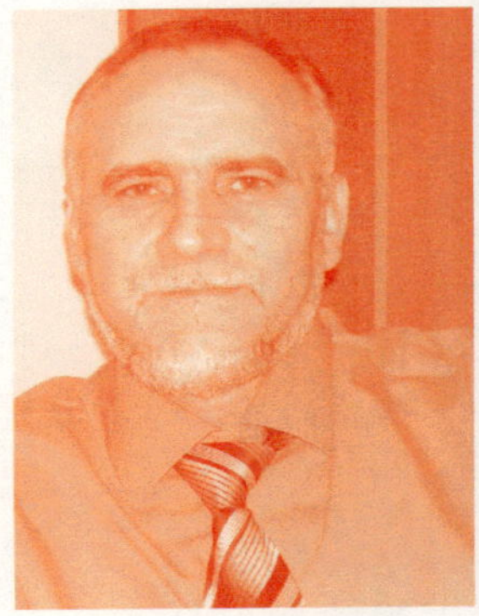
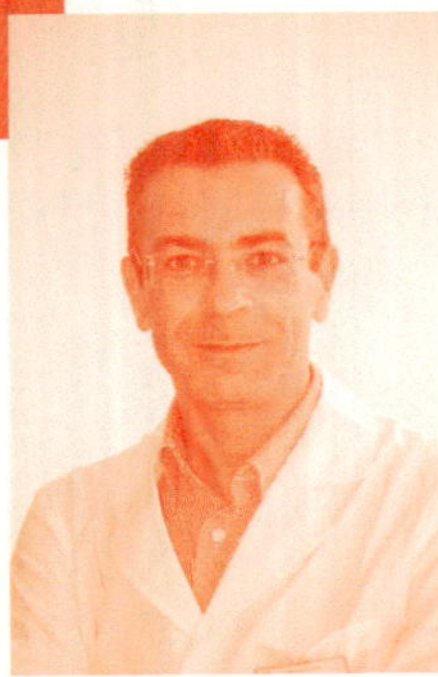
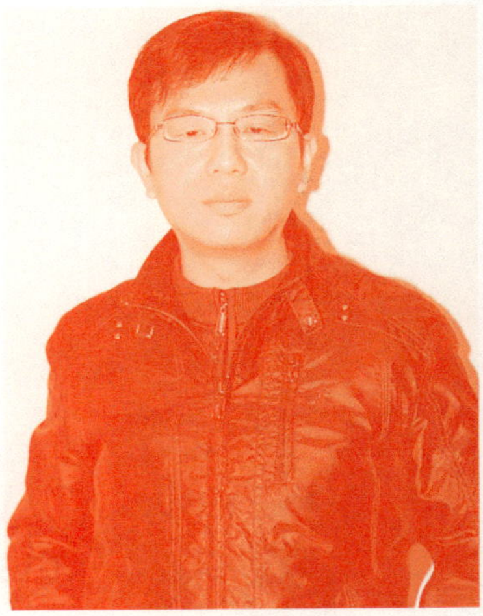
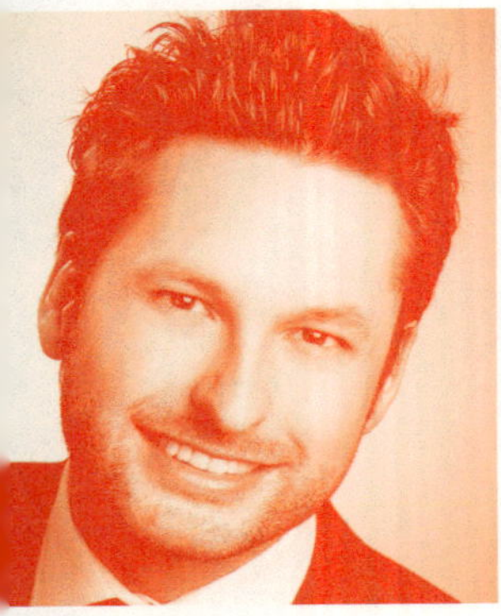
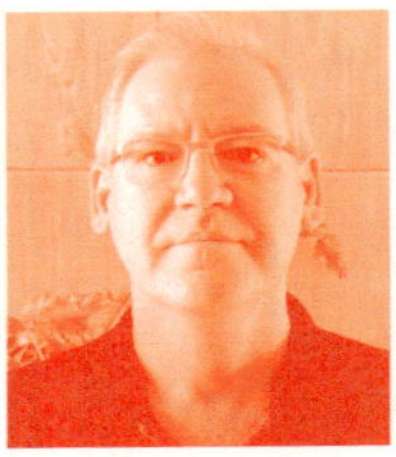

IntechOpen

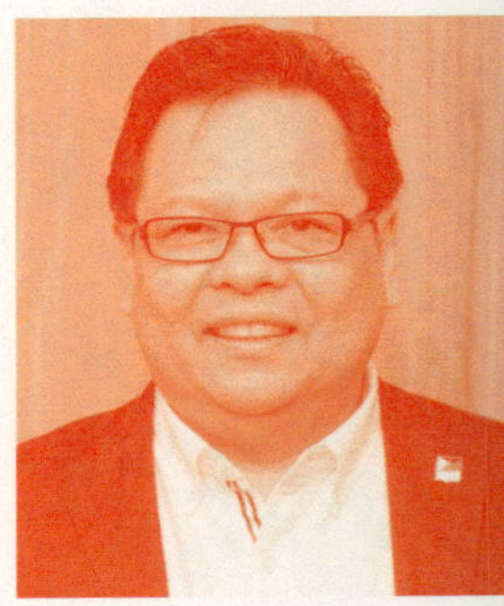
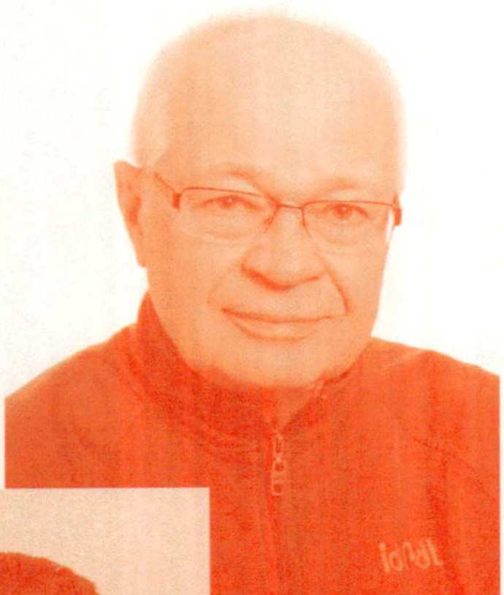
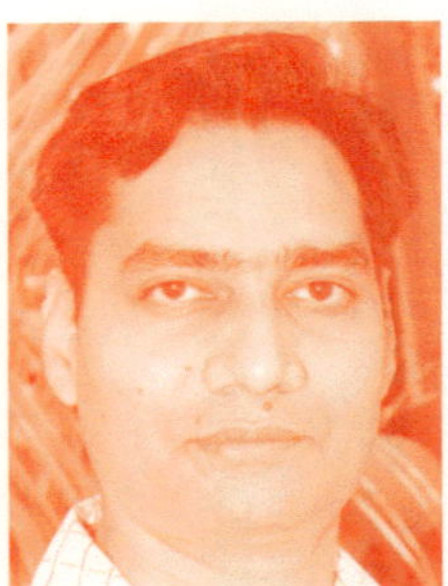
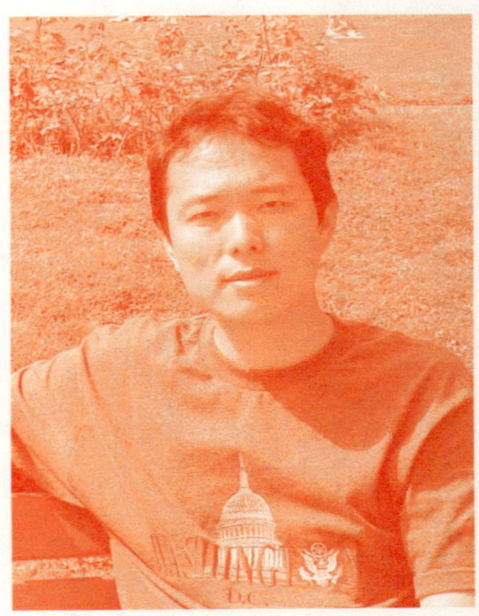
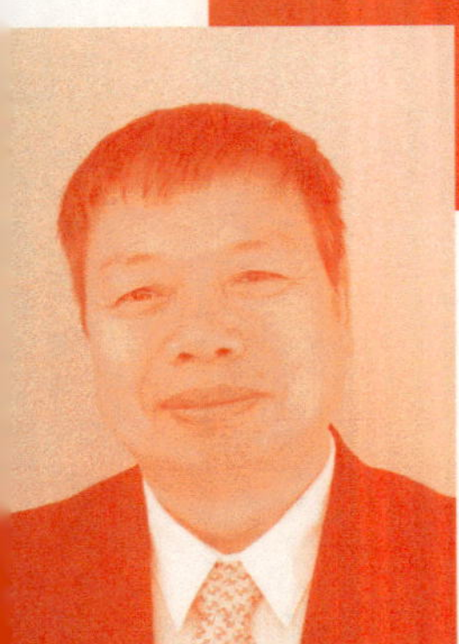
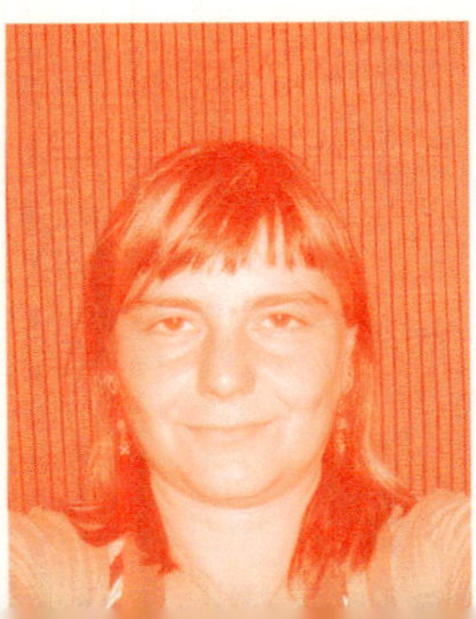

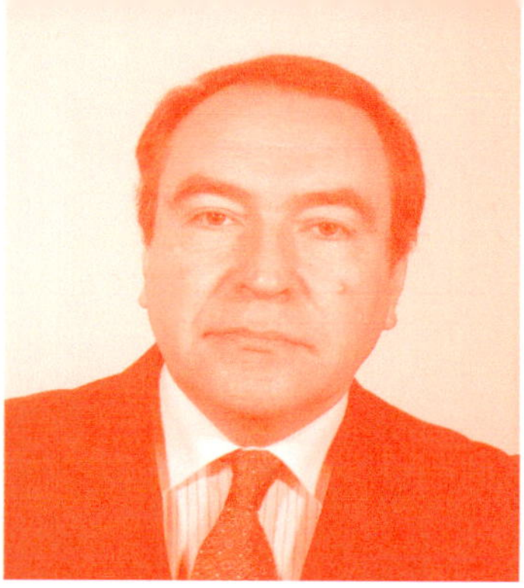
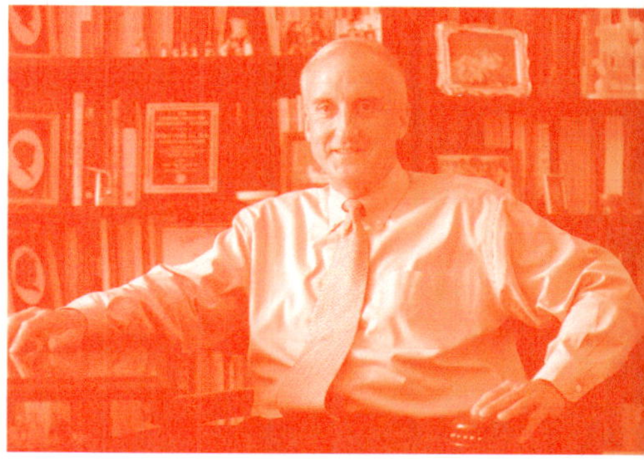
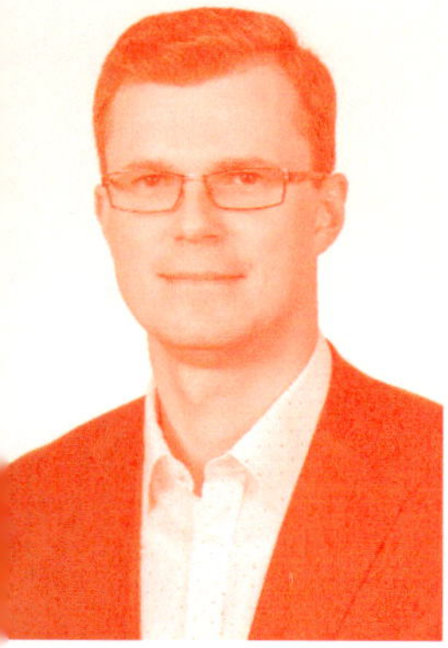
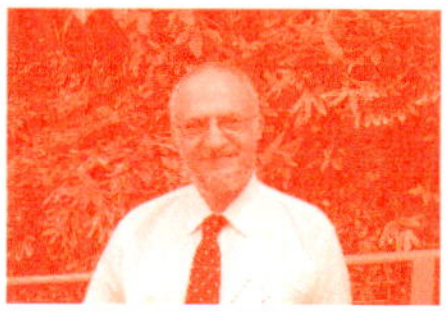
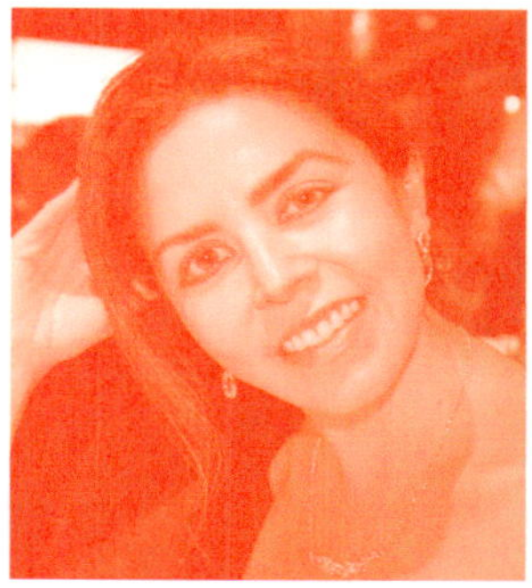

Supporting open minds since 2005

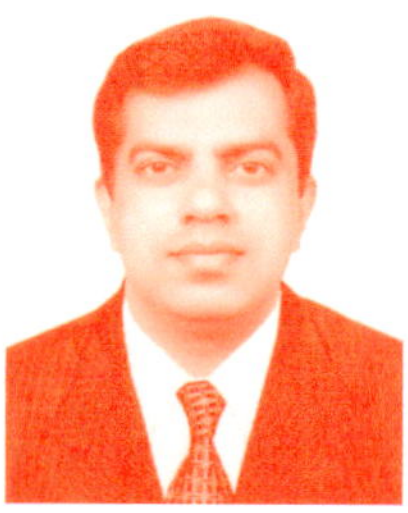
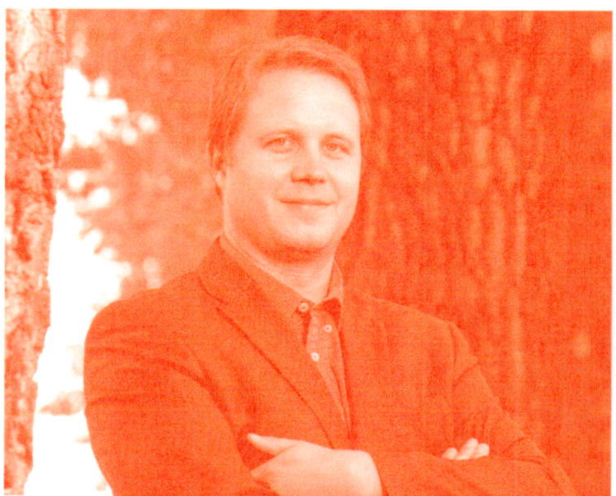
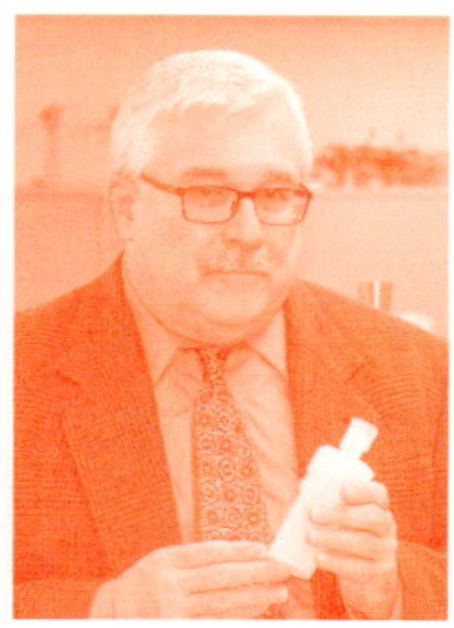
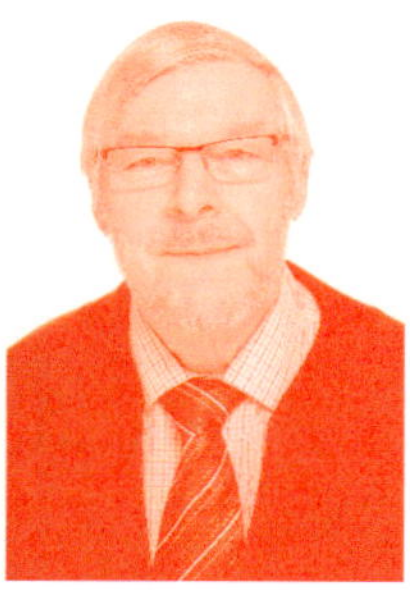
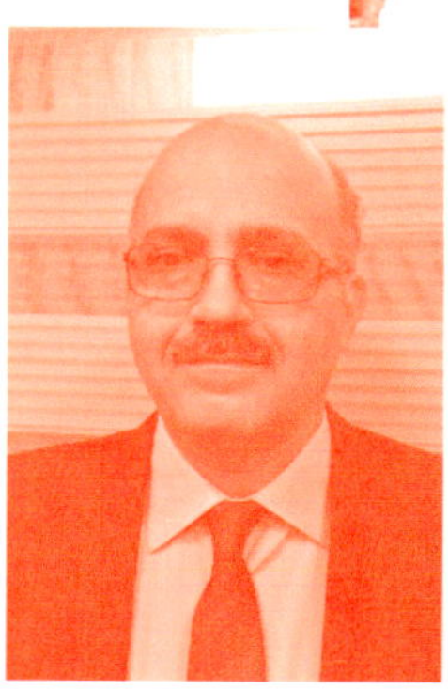
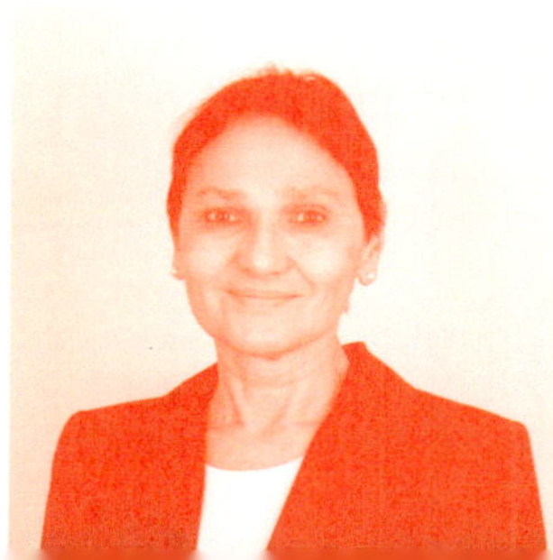
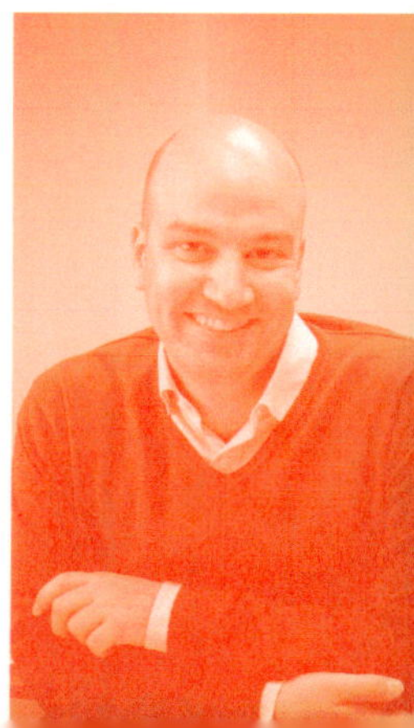

Frontiers in Ophthalmology and Ocular Imaging
http://dx.doi.org/10.5772/intechopen.75372
Edited by Alireza Ziaei

Contributors
Lawan Abdu, Ahmed Alnagdy, Adnan Saleem, Baris Komur, Shamim Saleha, Shaista Zafar, Kashif Rahim, Inayat Ullah Khan, Muhammad Yasin, Muhammad Dawood, Hind Alkatan, Tariq Al-Zahem, Norah Alkheraiji

First published in London, United Kingdom, 2019 by IntechOpen
IntechOpen is the global imprint of INTECHOPEN LIMITED, registered in England and Wales, registration number: 11086078, The Shard, 25th floor, 32 London Bridge Street
London, SE19SG - United Kingdom
Printed in Croatia

British Library Cataloguing-in-Publication Data
A catalogue record for this book is available from the British Library

Additional hard and PDF copies can be obtained from orders@intechopen.com

Frontiers in Ophthalmology and Ocular Imaging
Edited by Alireza Ziaei
p. cm.
Print ISBN 978-1-83880-806-8
Online ISBN 978-1-83880-807-5
eBook (PDF) ISBN 978-1-83880-808-2

For EU product safety concerns:
IN TECH d.o.o., Prolaz Marije Krucifikse Kozulić 3, 51000 Rijeka, Croatia, info@intechopen.com or visit our website at intechopen.com.

Meet the editor

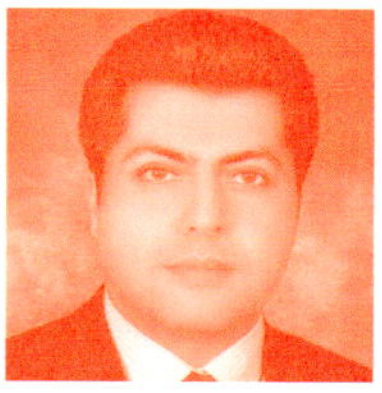

Dr. Alireza Ziaei, MD, is a physician-scientist at Harvard Medical School in Boston, USA. He is a recipient of numerous awards, including the National Excellent Researcher Award, National Young Investigator Award, and Science Excellence Prize. His main areas of interest are medical image processing and analysis, molecular base of ophthalmic disease and pathology pathways, radiological detection, and image-guided therapy. He has considerable experience in biomedical research at Schepens Eye Research Institute, Massachusetts Eye and Ear, with a focus on corneal and ocular surface diseases, and at National Center for Image-Guided Therapy, Brain Tumor Consortium, and BCH Neuroimaging Center on radiological cancer detection at Harvard BWH/BCH hospitals. Dr. Ziaei's seminal work has been recognized several times. He has published and presented numerous articles in highly ranked peer-reviewed journals and conferences worldwide. Dr. Ziaei has been a scientific member of ARVO, AAO, ISMRM, RSNA, ISBMT, TFOS, and MMS. He serves as an executive editor, an editorial board member, and a scientific reviewer of reputed journals and scientific societies, including *Nature International Journal of Science*, *Investigative Ophthalmology & Visual Science (IOVS)*, *American Journal of Ophthalmology (AJO)*, *The Journal of Clinical & Experimental Ophthalmology*, *The Journal of Cell Biology*, and *The Journal of Abdominal Radiology*.

Contents

Preface

There's likely a good reason for you to read an article in ophthalmology. A career in medicine includes the love of science and personal dedication. At some point in your medical or academic career, you decided to work in a field that improves people's health, an understandable choice—the restoring of any amount of vision to an individual can profoundly improve a person's quality of life. Blindness is an important symptom of many eye disorders. The estimated cost of global vision loss today is $3 trillion (USD). Science and research have always been crucial to furthering our understanding of ophthalmic conditions and their treatment and prevention. Ophthalmology researches have resulted in major advancements in medical science and ophthalmic practice. Discoveries made in various fields including genetics, immunology, and ocular biology have reshaped the foundations of ophthalmology and formed many new paradigms for the repair, regeneration, and rehabilitation of countless disorders. Enough has been achieved already to make it clear that this field has already produced some fundamental insights and has enormous possibilities for improving human health.

Imagination is the key to any discovery, and its presence in the science to improve eyesight and vision is no exception. Progress in vision science is racing forward, spurred on by a host of exciting new research discoveries and the efforts of scientists. And the moment the solution to a problem has societal relevance, it is no longer acceptable to restrict the tools used to find the answer to a single field. The complementary nature of many of the researches generates a highly interactive and collaborative environment that promotes the development of novel approaches to address fundamental questions. In the world today, scientists have accomplished that which previously was the domain of miracle workers. I have been inspired by my patients, colleagues, and mentors many times during my career. I have learned that one shining star on a dark night can help a person reach his or her destination. "Hope" is what you and your patient should never lose. I was trilled to be guided by a superb mentor, the late Dr. Ali Asghar Khodadoust, the legend of ophthalmology and a pioneer of eye research, with his deeply serene smile, who always believed, "As long as it is Rooted in the water, there is a Hope to fruit!"

A major challenge for the next decade will be to translate these advances into identifying the design and testing of novel approaches for disease treatments. But, yes ... the future is now! This book is a collection of reviewed and relevant research chapters, which intends to provide readers with a comprehensive overview of the latest and most advanced findings in several aspects of ophthalmology, ophthalmic pathology, ocular imaging, and certain treatment and surgical strategies. It is an excellent, well-integrated review of treatment options in eye disease that aims at providing a thorough overview of the recent developments written by international authors; it can be used as an important reference for clinically oriented ophthalmologists and scientists. Here are many valuable contributions from physicians and scientists who are experts in the field, and I thank all the contributors for their kind efforts in the preparation of this book.

Alireza Ziaei, MD
Harvard Medical School,
Boston, Massachusetts, USA

Chapter 1

Corneal Dystrophies and Degenerations

Hind Alkatan, Norah Alkheraiji and Tariq Alzahem

Abstract

The cornea is a complex structure with complex functions aiming to protect the internal ocular tissues and transmit and refract the coming light rays. Corneal dystrophies are a group of relatively infrequent genetic corneal disorders in which an abnormal material accumulates in the cornea causing variable loss of its clarity. On the other hand, corneal degenerations are more common and usually result from physiologic changes related to aging, particular disease, or long-standing environmental insults to the cornea. Ectatic corneal disorders are usually characterized by bilateral loss of corneal biomechanical strength leading to progressive thinning and bulging of the cornea with resultant astigmatism and decreased visual acuity. In this chapter, we will describe the basic embryological, anatomical, histologic, and physiological features of the cornea. Then, we will go over the clinical, histopathologic, medical, and surgical aspects of dystrophic, degenerative, and ectatic corneal disorders.

Keywords: cornea, physiology, embryology, anatomy, histopathology, genetic, classification, epidemiology, clinical, topography, dystrophy, degeneration, ectasia, keratoconus, keratopathy, keratoplasty

1. Introduction

The wall of the eye globe is composed of the cornea and the sclera. The latter covers the posterior four-fifths of the globe with anterior and posterior openings for the cornea and the optic nerve, respectively. The cornea is the most anterior part of the globe and is normally optically clear. A healthy overlying tear film is important for the optimal function of the cornea and the esthetic wellness of the ocular surface.

The cornea is a complex structure that is responsible for protection and about three-quarters of the optical power of the natural eye with the remainder coming from the crystalline lens. The normal cornea is devoid of blood vessels to insure optimal transmission of light rays. Oxygen and nutrients are supplied, and metabolic products are eliminated primarily through the tear film anteriorly and aqueous humor posteriorly. The cornea is one of the most densely innervated tissues in the body. Thus, traumatic corneal abrasions, bacterial keratitis, and bullous keratopathy are associated with severe pain, tearing, and photophobia. The corneal nerve plexuses are supplied by the first division (ophthalmic nerve) of the fifth cranial nerve (trigeminal nerve) [1].

Corneal dystrophies are defined as a group of slowly progressive, usually inherited, bilateral, and symmetric corneal opacifying disorders that might be associated with variable degrees of decreased vision and discomfort. Typically, they are not linked to environmental or systemic factors. Nevertheless, there are exceptions to each portion of the corneal dystrophies' definition, as some dystrophies are unilateral and asymmetric and have no recognizable heredity and have associated systemic findings [2]. Based on the cellular origin of corneal dystrophy, a modified anatomic classification is proposed consisting of epithelial and subepithelial, epithelial-stromal, stromal, and endothelial dystrophies [3].

Degenerations generally result from steady deterioration of the tissues that was previously normal with subsequent loss of their functional activity. Corneal degenerations are characterized by the deposition of a specific material, stromal thinning, and vascularization. They are not hereditary and can be unilateral. The cornea may undergo changes associated with ultraviolet light stimulation and oxidative stress that are thought to be responsible for the progression of degenerative processes [4, 5].

Corneal ectasia refers to a group of noninflammatory conditions characterized by bilateral loss of corneal biomechanical strength leading to progressive thinning and bulging of the cornea with resultant irregular astigmatism and decreased visual acuity. Examples include keratoconus, post laser-assisted in situ keratomileusis (LASIK) ectasia, pellucid marginal degeneration, and keratoglobus [1].

We will start this chapter by describing the basic sciences of the normal human cornea including embryological, anatomical, histologic, and physiological features of the cornea with mentioning selected related functional aspects. Later, we will discuss the most important corneal dystrophies, degenerations, and ectasia from clinical, histopathologic, and management points of view.

2. The basic sciences of the cornea

2.1 Corneal embryology

Corneal development and differentiation are the last in the well-organized series of ocular tissue formation. Thus, normal corneal development depends on normal development of the lens and optic cup. The corneal epithelium is derived from the surface ectoderm, while the corneal stroma, including Bowman's layer, and endothelium are derived from the neural crest cells. The Descemet's membrane is synthesized by endothelial cells and acts as the basement membrane of the corneal endothelium [6, 7].

The corneal development begins on the 22nd day of gestation as the surface ectoderm, the primordium of the corneal epithelium, and can be identified at the start of the 6th week of intrauterine age [8]. The neural crest cells come in three distinct waves. The first wave, in the 7th week, migrates between the primitive corneal epithelium and the lens epithelium to form the corneal endothelium. The second wave migrates to the area situated between the future corneal endothelium and the corneal epithelium and gives rise to keratocytes, the cells of the corneal stroma. The third wave of neural crest cells is located in the primitive anterior chamber to form the iris stroma [9–12].

Keratan sulfate is a proteoglycan that is produced by keratocytes and can be demonstrated at the 8th week of gestation. It is present in keratocytes and endothelial cells but not the epithelial cells [13–15]. The early corneal epithelium is composed of two layers, apical and basal layers. The outer (apical) cells are cuboidal without microvilli and are joined together by junctional complexes: zonula occludens and zonula adherens. They are connected to the basal cell by desmosomes [16]. The epithelium increases to three cell layers at 10-day postpartum and continues to thicken until reaching the adult thickness of about six layers by the 4th week of life [17].

2.2 Corneal anatomy, histology, and physiology

2.2.1 Corneoscleral limbus

The corneal limbus is simply described as the transition zone between the peripheral corneal margin and the anterior sclera. Its width is approximately 1–1.5 mm. One of the important characteristics of the limbus is that it contains the corneal stem cells detected in the basal cell layer. The limbus can be defined from histological, pathological, and surgical points of view.

From histological aspects, the anterior margin of the limbus is bounded by a line connecting the peripheral termination of Bowman's layer from the corneal epithelial side and the peripheral termination of Descemet's membrane, known as Schwalbe line, from the endothelial side. The peripheral margin is bordered by the scleral spur. From pathologists' point of view, a vertical line that is perpendicular to the scleral spur was added to define the peripheral margin [18]. Surgeons divide the limbus into two zones: a central blue zone and a peripheral concentric white zone. The area containing Bowman' layer and Descemet's membrane is seen as blue. The trabecular meshwork is located under the white zone [19].

2.2.2 Corneal anatomy

The cornea is the round transparent portion of the eyeball. It is the strongest refractive component of the optical system of the eye. To maintain its transparency, the normal cornea is avascular, relatively acellular, and relatively dehydrated with extraordinary organization of the stromal collagen lamellae. The diameter of the cornea measures 11–12 mm in horizontal meridian and 10–11 in vertical meridian. The average central thickness of the cornea is 520 and 650 μm peripherally. The corneal stroma is 78% water. This percentage is controlled by an intact epithelium and a normally functioning endothelial pump. The refractive index of the cornea is 1.376 [18].

In the following subsections, we will describe the histology and physiology of different layers of the cornea from the front to the back: epithelium, Bowman's layer, stroma, Descemet's membrane, and endothelium.

2.2.3 Corneal epithelium

As previously mentioned, the corneal epithelium is derived from the embryonic surface ectoderm and lies on the outer surface of the cornea. The epithelium is composed of 5–6 layers of nonkeratinized stratified squamous epithelium overlying a single layer of basal cells. It is 50 μm thick. Complete renewal of the epithelial cells occurs in 7–10 days. Three distinct layers of epithelial cells are identified: superficial flattened cells, middle wing cells, and deep basal cells [18].

The superficial and the wing cells differentiate from the basal cells. There are approximately 6000 basal cells/mm^2 in a normal cornea. They are derived from the corneal limbal stem cells. The new cells migrate from the limbus in a centripetal fashion at a speed of approximately 120 μm/week. Gab junctions serve to provide communication channels between basal cells. A basal lamina that is 50 nm thick, and is composed of type IV collagen, is actively secreted by the basal cells. The cells are attached to the underlying basal lamina via hemidesmosomes. Recurrent epithelial erosions, seen in patients with epithelial basement membrane dystrophy (EBMD), are caused by alteration of hemidesmosomes [18].

On the top of basal cells are 2–3 cell layers of wing cells. They resemble wings in cross section. Wing cells are joined together by zonulae occludentes forming a semipermeable membrane preventing components of the tear film from gaining entry to the corneal stroma. The superficial layer is composed of 2–3 rows of flattened cells. They shed in the tear film and are replenished by other cells. Microplicae and microvilli are observed on the apical surface of the superficial cells. Epithelial cells are attached to each other by desmosomes. Topical anesthetic abuse causes a decline in the number of desmosomes with resultant impaired healing [20].

2.2.4 Bowman's layer

Bowman's layer represents the most anterior part of the stroma and lies directly posterior to the basal lamina of the corneal epithelium. Bowman's layer is not considered a true membrane and does not stain with periodic acid-Schiff (PAS). It is 8–12 μm thick and composed of type I and type V collagen. After injury, Bowman's layer does not regenerate and, thus, a scar will form. In contrast to the stroma, the collagen lamellae are smaller and randomly organized [18].

Bowman's layer is critical in supporting the corneal biomechanics through its stiff and strong nature. Weakening of this layer can result in ectatic corneal disorders, such as keratoconus, due to loss of the biomechanical support [21].

2.2.5 Corneal stroma

The corneal stroma is derived from the neural crest cells. It constitutes around 90–95% of the corneal thickness. Numerically, the central corneal thickness measures about 0.52 mm and thickens to 0.65 mm in the periphery. It has corneal stromal collagen lamellae, 200–250 lamellae that are arranged parallel to the surface of the cornea. They are predominantly made from type I and type V collagens. Keratan sulfate and dermatan sulfate are the primary proteoglycans of the stroma. These proteoglycans are located between the lamellae maintaining a constant interlamellar distance, an important factor in eliminating light scatter and, thus, a clear cornea [18]. In 2013, an acellular layer measuring approximately 10 μm in the posterior stroma, named the pre-Descemet's layer (or Dua's layer), was introduced [22].

There are approximately 2.4 million keratocytes in the corneal stroma scattered in between the lamellae. They synthesize collagen and proteoglycans. Keratocytes are abundant in mitochondria, rough endoplasmic reticulum, and Golgi apparatuses. The plasma membranes are fenestrated, and they communicate via gab junctions. There is a documented decline in the cell density associated with age [18].

The anterior part of the stroma is typically drier than the posterior part. This is caused by the drying effect of the atmosphere anteriorly and the wetting effect of the aqueous humor posteriorly. An enlarged spacing between the lamellae, as in cases of corneal stromal edema from endothelial injury, will result in hazy cornea and decreased visual acuity [18].

2.2.6 Descemet's membrane (DM)

Descemet's membrane is a true basement membrane, for corneal endothelium, that is PAS positive. The thickness of DM varies according to the age of the individual. It is continuously secreted by the endothelium through life. In newborns, it measures about 2–4 μm in thickness and reaches to 10–12 μm in adults [18].

Histologically, DM has two layers: an anterior banded layer produced during fetal life and a posterior non-banded layer produced after birth. It is made of type IV collagen, laminin, and fibronectin [18].

DM provides support and adhesion to endothelial cells. Under pathologic conditions, it works as a biologic barrier to the phagocytic, toxic, and enzymatic degradation. Notably, DM is weakly attached to the overlying stroma, or pre-Descemet's layer, and can be surgically dissected as one piece (Descemetorrhexis) [18].

2.2.7 Corneal endothelium

The corneal endothelium is the innermost layer of the cornea. It is about 4–6 μm thick. As mentioned earlier, the endothelium originates from neural crest cells. The cells cannot be replenished if lost. There are about 500,000 endothelial cells covering the posterior surface of the cornea with a density of 3000 cells/mm^2. There is approximately 0.6% endothelial cell loss per year, and this rate increases significantly after traumatic, iatrogenic, inflammatory, or infectious conditions affecting the endothelium. The most common normal cell shape is hexagonal with minimal polymegathism and pleomorphism [18].

To maintain the corneal clarity, the endothelium works as a barrier and as a metabolic pump. Endothelial cells are linked together by interdigitations and focal tight junctions. They communicate via gab junctions. Some nutrients are allowed to pass paracellularly to the remaining corneal layers indicating a semipermeable nature of the endothelial cell layer [18].

The corneal endothelium is a highly active tissue. This is evident by the presence of numerous mitochondria, the prominent endoplasmic reticulum, ribosomes, and Golgi apparatus. The fluid is pumped out of the corneal stroma into the anterior chamber via pinocytic vesicles [18].

Hassall-Henle bodies, or peripheral cornea guttae, are considered a natural aging process in which small excrescences are observed in the peripheral part of Descemet's membrane. They denote focal areas of thickening of Descemet's membrane. On the other hand, central cornea guttae are pathologic in nature and are associated with progressive corneal stromal and epithelial edema as in patients with Fuchs' endothelial dystrophy [18].

3. Corneal dystrophies

Generally, corneal dystrophies are defined as a group of progressive, inherited, mostly bilateral, and symmetric, variable corneal opacifying disorders, which are usually not related to environmental or systemic conditions. The can be associated with blurred vision and ocular discomfort. Their onset is usually early in life but they manifest later clinically. They are slowly progressive and become more prominent with age. There are exceptions to the corneal dystrophies definition: some dystrophies are unilateral or bilateral asymmetric, some have no obvious heredity, and some have related systemic abnormalities [1, 2].

In 2015, the International Committee on the Classification of Corneal Dystrophies (IC3D) proposed a modified anatomic classification on the basis of the cellular origin of the corneal dystrophies consisting of [3]:

1. Epithelial and subepithelial dystrophies

2. Epithelial-stromal transforming growth factor β-induced gene (TGFBI) dystrophies

3. Stromal dystrophies

4. Endothelial dystrophies

An evidence-based category system was suggested to indicate the level of evidence that supports the existence of a given corneal dystrophy. In this system, each dystrophy is organized according to the clinical phenotype, with a template summarizing genetic, clinical, and pathologic information. The system is upgradable and can be retrieved at www.corneasociety.org. The categories are as follows [23]:

Category 1 (C1): a well-defined corneal dystrophy in which the gene has been mapped and identified and the specific mutations are known.

Category 2 (C2): a well-defined corneal dystrophy that has been mapped to one or more specific chromosomal loci, but the gene(s) remains to be identified.

Category 3 (C3): a well-defined corneal dystrophy in which the disorder has not yet been mapped to a chromosomal locus.

Category 4 (C4): this category is reserved for a suspected, new, or previously documented corneal dystrophy, although the evidence for it, being a distinct entity, is not yet convincing.

In the following subsections, we will describe the clinical, genetic, and histopathologic characteristics of the common corneal dystrophies from anterior to posterior: epithelial and subepithelial, epithelial-stromal (TGFBI), stromal, and endothelial dystrophies.

3.1 Epithelial and subepithelial corneal dystrophies

The included dystrophies are:

1. Epithelial basement membrane dystrophy (EBMD)

2. Epithelial recurrent erosion dystrophies (EREDs)—Franceschetti corneal dystrophy (FRCD), Dystrophia smolandiensis (DS), and Dystrophia helsinglandica

3. Subepithelial mucinous corneal dystrophy (SMCD)

4. Meesmann corneal dystrophy (MECD)

5. Lisch epithelial corneal dystrophy (LECD)

6. Gelatinous drop-like corneal dystrophy (GDLD)

3.1.1 Epithelial basement membrane dystrophy (EBMD)

EBMD, also known as map-dot-fingerprint dystrophy [24], Cogan's microcystic epithelial dystrophy [25], and anterior basement membrane dystrophy, is the most common anterior corneal dystrophy. It can reach up to 70% in individuals above the age of 50 years and is found to be infrequent in the pediatric population [26]. It was found to be more common in females [27].

Inheritance: mostly sporadic with familial cases have been reported. Thus, they are thought to be degenerative or caused by previous trauma.

Genetic locus and gene: 5q31. One report has identified TGFBI in two families.

Category: most cases are sporadic. C1 in rare cases.

Onset: usually in the second decade.

Symptoms: it maybe asymptomatic or associated with recurrent epithelial erosions in 10% of patients due to poor adhesion of basal epithelial cells to the basal

DOI: http://dx.doi.org/10.5772/intechopen.84426

laminar material. Irregular astigmatism might cause decreased vision and monocular diplopia. The severity of pathology can fluctuate with time.

Signs: can be isolated or combined and unilateral or bilateral.

- Maps: central or paracentral thickened, scalloped, circumscribed borders resembling coastlines, associated with faint haze.
- Fingerprints: paracentral, hair-like, curvilinear concentric lines, best visualized with retro-illumination.
- Dots: central, round or oval, non-staining, intraepithelial opacities. These lesions contain debris of degenerated epithelial cells.
- Bleb pattern: subepithelial bleb or cobble stone-like pattern, best seen by retro-illumination.

Histopathology:

- Maps: thickened intraepithelial, multilamellar, basement membrane.
- Fingerprints: intraepithelial extensions of basement membrane that are rib-like.
- Dots: intraepithelial cyst-like lesions containing degenerated cytoplasmic debris.
- Bleb pattern: subepithelial fibrillo-granular material accumulation.
- Bowman's layer is not affected.

Management: in asymptomatic cases no intervention is required. When symptoms occur, the frequent use of lubricants is recommended (preferably preservative-free lubricants). Hypertonic drops (i.e., sodium chloride 3–5%) during the daytime and an ointment at night can be helpful. Topical antibiotics are needed in cases where there are erosions. Cautious wear of a bandage contact lens may help in providing comfort and healing. In severe cases, debridement of the epithelial surface might be needed, and, in some cases, a phototherapeutic keratectomy (PTK) might be helpful.

3.1.2 Epithelial recurrent erosion dystrophies (EREDs)

Inheritance: autosomal dominant.

Variants:

- Franceschetti corneal dystrophy (FRCD)
- Dystrophia smolandiensis (DS)
- Dystrophia helsinglandica (DH)

Genetic locus and gene: unknown.

Category: C3.

Onset: childhood.

Symptoms: recurrent epithelial erosion attacks that start in childhood and continue in adulthood. The attacks are usually nocturnal. Corneal opacification, which may be visually significant if located centrally, occurs in about half of the cases. Painful erosive episodes usually decrease with age.

Signs: repeated epithelial erosions lasting up to 7 days in duration. Typically, no signs can be detected after healing of the attack. However, central subepithelial opacities, subepithelial fibrosis, or corneal keloids may develop later in life.

Histopathology: the basal epithelial cells are irregular with distended intercellular spaces. Intracellular and intercellular Alcian blue-positive deposits are present. Bowman's layer is partial or completely destructed. Avascular pannus is between the basal epithelium and the Bowman layer [3].

Management: in asymptomatic patients, treatment is not required. Recurrent erosive episodes are treated as for recurrent epithelial erosions. Epithelial debridement may be necessary in patient with irregular astigmatism.

3.1.3 Subepithelial mucinous corneal dystrophy (SMCD)

Inheritance: mostly autosomal dominant.

Genetic locus and gene: unknown.

Category: C4.

Onset: early childhood.

Symptoms: painful epithelial erosions that might decrease in frequency with age. The vision tends to deteriorate with time.

Signs: subepithelial haze denser in the center.

Histopathology: subepithelial band of eosinophilic, periodic acid-Schiff (PAS)-positive, Alcian blue-positive, hyaluronidase-sensitive material is present anterior to the Bowman layer [3].

Management: recurrent erosive episodes are treated as for recurrent epithelial erosions.

3.1.4 Meesmann corneal dystrophy (MECD)

MECD is also known as Meesmann-Wilke syndrome and Meesmann's juvenile epithelial corneal dystrophy [28, 29].

Inheritance: mostly autosomal dominant.

Variant: stocker-Holt variant.

Genetic locus and gene: 2 loci and 2 genes.

- Locus 12q13 (KRT3 gene)
- Locus 17q12 (KRT12 gene) in Stocker-Holt variant

Category: C1.

Onset: usually in the first decade.

Symptoms: most patients are asymptomatic. Glare, photophobia, decreased vision, or recurrent epithelial erosions may occur. It is slowly progressive or even nonprogressive. Patients affected with Stocker-Holt variant show more severe signs and symptoms with earlier onset.

Signs: bilateral and symmetric numerous central and peripheral intraepithelial vesicles most dense in the interpalpebral area. Gray opacities usually having a distinct border with some areas being spared. Microcysts are seen in about 80% of corneas and are more evident with retro-illumination. These cysts coalesce resulting in refractile linear opacities. Mild corneal thinning or reduced sensation may occur. In patients with Stocker-Holt variant, diffuse grayish punctate superficial opacities that stain with fluorescein are observed.

Histopathology: the epithelium is thickened and disorganized exhibiting intraepithelial cysts filled with PAS-positive cellular debris. There is a multilaminar, thickened basement membrane extending into the basal epithelium. Bowman's layer and corneal stroma that remain are not affected [3].

Management: in symptomatic cases, strategies for relief of the epithelial erosions include topical antibiotics to protect against infection, heavy lubrication, and contact lens application. In more severe cases, epithelial debridement and corneal keratoplasty are considered [30].

3.1.5 Lisch epithelial corneal dystrophy (LECD)

History: Lisch epithelial corneal dystrophy (LECD) was first described in 1992 in five family members and three unrelated individuals who presented with unilateral or bilateral bands of grayish granular opacifications on the cornea [31].

Inheritance: X-chromosomal dominant.

Genetic locus and gene: Xp22.3, the gene is unknown.

Category: C2.

Onset: childhood.

Symptoms: asymptomatic if the dystrophy is not involving the pupillary axis. Slowly progressive with decreased visual acuity if the corneal center is involved.

Signs: gray opacities that come in different patterns including band-shaped, radial, feathery, and whorl-like. Multiple clear cysts are seen with indirect illumination resembling MECD. However, the difference is in the molecular genetics.

Histopathology: PAS-positive vacuolated cells are present in the epithelial surface [3].

Management: treatment only if the individual is symptomatic with heavy lubrication. In some cases, debridement might be helpful. Phototherapeutic keratectomy (PTK) can be beneficial in some cases [32].

3.1.6 Gelatinous drop-like corneal dystrophy (GDLD)

GDLD was first described by Nakaizumi (1914) [33]. It was found to be more common in Japan.

Inheritance: autosomal recessive.

Genetic locus and gene: 1p32, tumor-associated calcium signal transducer 2 (TACSTD2).

Category: C1.

Onset: during the first 2 decades.

Symptoms: blurred vision, photophobia, foreign body sensation, and tearing.

Signs: subepithelial lesions may look like band keratopathy initially. Mulberry configuration of nodules that stain with fluorescein can occur. This configuration indicates epithelial hyperpermeability. Vascularization and stromal scarring are seen later in the course of the disease.

Histopathology: amyloid deposits in the subepithelial and stromal [3].

Management: treatment for symptomatic cases includes heavy lubrication. Superficial keratectomy or keratoplasty can be helpful when there is visual impairment. Recurrence is common following superficial keratectomy, lamellar keratoplasty, and penetrating keratoplasty [34].

3.2 Epithelial-stromal TGFBI dystrophies

The included dystrophies are:

1. Reis-Bücklers corneal dystrophy (RBCD)

2. Thiel-Behnke corneal dystrophy (TBCD)

3. Lattice corneal dystrophy, type 1 (LCD1)

4. Granular corneal dystrophy, type 1 (GCD1)

5. Granular corneal dystrophy, type 2 (GCD2)

3.2.1 Reis-Bucklers corneal dystrophy (RBCD)

RBCD was first described in 1917. It is also known as geographic corneal dystrophy of Weidle, superficial granular corneal dystrophy, atypical granular corneal dystrophy, granular corneal dystrophy type 3, and anterior limiting membrane dystrophy type 1 [35].

Inheritance: autosomal dominant.

Genetic locus and gene: 5q31, transforming growth factor β-induced gene (TGFBI).

Category: C1.

Onset: during the first decade of life.

Symptoms: blurred vision and recurrent corneal epithelial erosions. It is slowly progressive. The frequency of recurrent corneal erosions tends to decline with age. It has a more aggressive course than Thiel-Behnke corneal dystrophy (TBCD). In addition, the diagnosis can be confused between RBCD and TBCD.

Signs: early in the course of the disease, there are varying densities of bilateral irregular geographic-like opacities with clear interruptions at the level of Bowman's layer and anterior stroma. They are discrete in early stages and become diffuse with deeper involvement. As the disease progresses, these fine reticular lesions coalesce to form a confluent gray whitish opacity that might affect vision as the surface becomes more irregular. At later stages, the corneal sensation is reduced, and ring-shaped (sometimes crescent-shaped) opacifications cover the central cornea and can extend to the mid-periphery. The most peripheral cornea remains clear.

Histopathology: granular sheet-like deposits replace Bowman's layer. These deposits stain red with Masson trichrome. The anterior, middle, and even posterior stroma can be involved in advanced cases. Electron microscopy is required to distinguish RBCD from TBCD. In RBCD, rod-shaped subepithelial bodies are seen, while curly fibers are characteristic for TBCD [3].

Management: treatment of corneal erosions is similar to that of other dystrophies. Phototherapeutic keratectomy (PTK) can be beneficial in some cases. In advanced corneal involvement, keratoplasty might be helpful.

3.2.2 Thiel-Behnke corneal dystrophy (TBCD)

TBCD is also known as corneal dystrophy of Bowman's layer type II, curly fibers corneal dystrophy, Waardenburg-Jonkers corneal dystrophy, and, most commonly, "honeycomb dystrophy." It was first described in 1967 [36–38].

Inheritance: autosomal dominant.

Genetic locus and gene: 5q31, TGFBI.

Category: C1.

Onset: during the first decade of life.

Symptoms: visual deterioration occurs later, and recurrent corneal epithelial erosions are less frequent than in RBCD. Slowly progressive corneal scarring is the main cause of decreased vision. The recurrence of corneal erosions decreases with time.

Signs: irregularly shaped scattered opacities and solitary flecks at the level of the Bowman's layer are present in the initial stages. Then, central honeycomb opacities are observed in the subepithelial area. As in patients with RBCD, corneal opacities can progress peripherally and to deeper stromal layers. Prominent corneal nerves can be seen. The corneal periphery remains clear even as the lesions progress. Corneal sensation might be affected. Reis-Buckler's dystrophy and Thiel-Behnke can be clinically distinguished by the minimal loss of corneal sensation and honeycomb opacity that occurs with Thiel-Behnke dystrophy [37, 39].

Histopathology: irregular thickening and thinning of the epithelial layer due to irregular underlying stroma with focal absence of the epithelial basement membrane. Wavy saw-toothed superficial fibro-cellular pannus replaces the Bowman's layer [3].

Management: treatment is indicated only in symptomatic cases. The episodes of recurrent erosion are treated like the previous dystrophies. Hypertonic drops and ointment may be beneficial. In some cases, debridement of the corneal epithelium may be necessary. Phototherapeutic keratectomy (PTK) can also help with recurrent erosions or superficial opacifications [37, 39]. Keratoplasty is reserved for deeper lesions, but the dystrophy may recur in the donor graft.

3.2.3 Lattice corneal dystrophy, type 1 (LCD1) and variants

Inheritance: autosomal dominant.

Variants: LCD (III, IIIA, I/IIIA, IV). Lattice corneal dystrophy type 2 (LCD2) is a misnomer and should be termed familial amyloidosis, Finnish type, or gelsolin type as suggested by the IC3D. LCD2 is also known as Meretoja syndrome.

Genetic locus and gene: 5q31, TGFBI.

Category: C1.

Onset: during the first two decades of life.

Symptoms: visual deterioration, discomfort, and pain. Recurrent attacks of corneal erosions occur early in the course of LCD1. Patients with progressive visual impairment are seen within the fourth decade.

Signs: central superficial fleck-like opacities are seen initially. By using retro-illumination technique, sparse peripheral lattice lines are visible initially in the superficial stroma (**Figure 1A**). Centrally located, superficial branching refractile lines resembling tree branches and round/ovoid whitish dots are also detected in the first decade (**Figure 1B**). Central and paracentral diffuse subepithelial haze develops alongside the lattice lines. They typically spare the limbus, Descemet's membrane, and endothelium. The average depth in the stroma is about 79 μm [40]. Reduction of visual acuity is caused by the progression of the stromal haze (**Figure 1C**). LCD1 may be asymmetric or even unilateral. Central thicker lattice lines are seen in variant LCD type IIIA, while LCD type IV is characterized by deeper deposits without epithelial erosion.

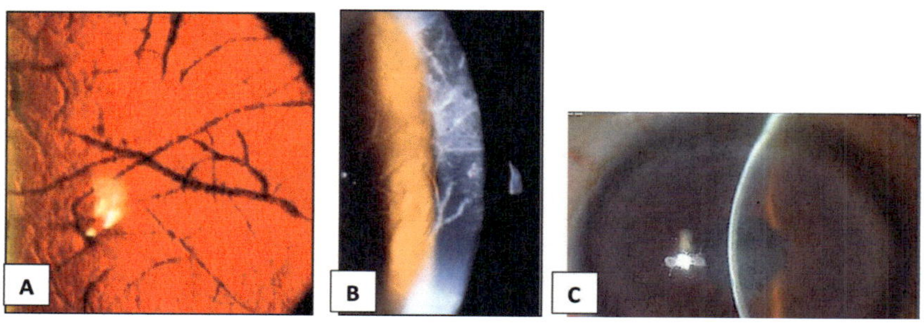

Figure 1.
(A) The appearance of the lattice deposits with retro-illumination, (B) slit lamp appearance of the lattice configuration of the stromal deposits in this type of dystrophy, and (C) clinical appearance of an advanced case of lattice dystrophy.

Histopathology: the corneal epithelium is atrophic with degenerative changes of basal epithelial cells. The Bowman's layer is disrupted or even absent. Subepithelial accumulation and stromal accumulation of amyloid deposits alter the architecture of corneal collagen lamellae (**Figure 2**). These deposits stain positive with Congo red and show birefringence with polarizing light (**Figure 3**) [41]. Metachromasia and fluorescence are demonstrated with crystal violet and thioflavin T staining, respectively. Descemet's membrane and the endothelium are normal [3].

Management: treatment is based on the symptoms and the depth of the deposits. Options might include phototherapeutic keratectomy (PTK) with anterior lesions and where there are recurrent corneal erosions, lamellar keratoplasty (LKP) and penetrating keratoplasty (PKP) for deeper lesions. Reports on recurrence after DLKP that was associated with incomplete removal of corneal stroma [42]. Overall, recurrence was reported to be earlier compared to macular and granular corneal dystrophies [43].

3.2.4 Granular corneal dystrophy, type 1 (classic) (GCD1)

Inheritance: autosomal dominant.
Genetic locus and gene: 5q31, TGFBI.
Category: C1.
Onset: early childhood.

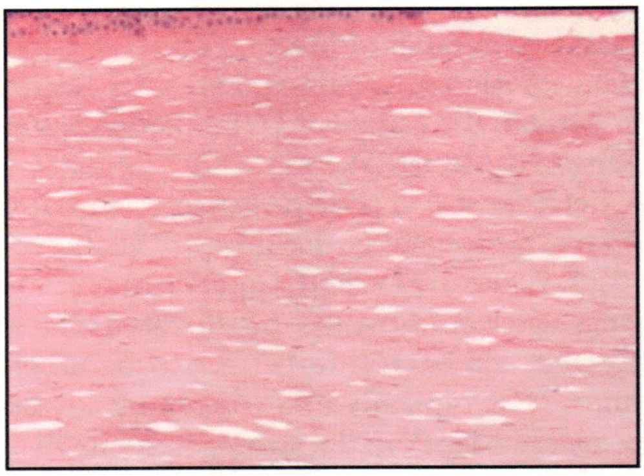

Figure 2.
The amyloid deposits within the stroma in lattice dystrophy (original magnification 200× hematoxylin & eosin).

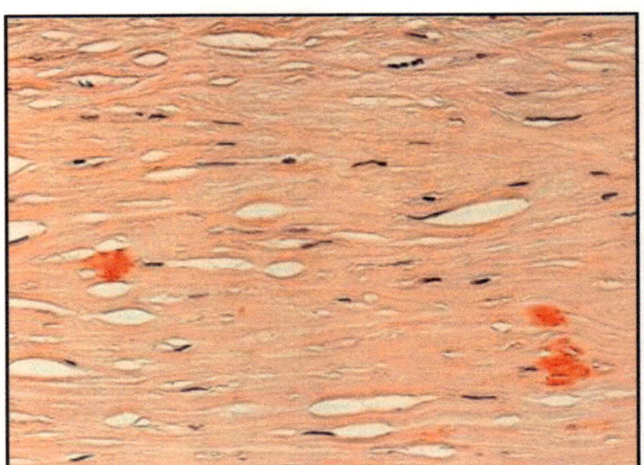

Figure 3.
The same amyloid deposits staining with Congo red stain (original magnification 400× Congo red).

Symptoms: patients usually complain of glare, photophobia, and recurrent erosions. Visual deterioration occurs as corneal opacification progresses with time as the opacities become more confluent.

Signs: initially, subepithelial verticillate-like opacities are evident by retro- and direct illumination. Later, there will be white well-defined granules with clear intervening stroma (**Figure 4**). Typically, opacities do not extend to the limbus. With age, granules extend deeper into the corneal stroma close to Descemet's membrane.

Histopathology: multiple stromal deposits may extend from deep epithelium to Descemet's membrane. Hyaline opacities stain with Masson trichrome (**Figure 5A** and **B**) [3, 41].

Management: treatment options if symptomatic include lubrication, hypertonic solution, and bandage contact lenses. Phototherapeutic keratectomy (PTK) and keratoplasty for deeper lesions. Recurrence occurred in all grafts within 4 years [44].

3.2.5 Granular corneal dystrophy, type 2 (GCD2)

Nomenclature: also called combined granular-lattice corneal dystrophy or Avellino corneal dystrophy. It was named after the Avellino region in Italy, where first cases have been reported.

Inheritance: autosomal dominant.

Genetic locus and gene: 5q31, TGFBI.

Category: C1.

Onset: in homozygous patients, the onset is in early childhood. Heterozygous patients present in late childhood.

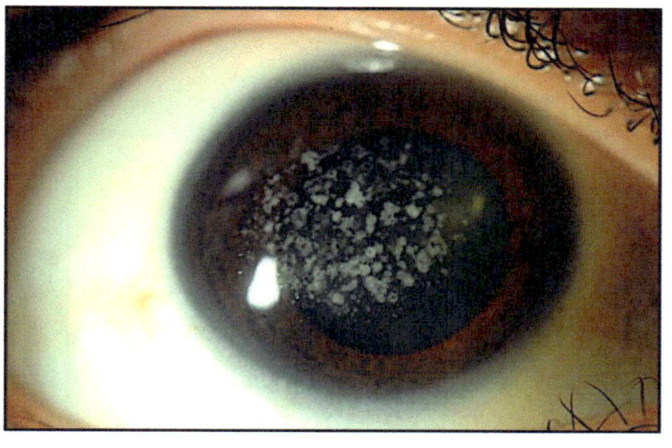

Figure 4.
The clinical appearance of granular dystrophy (courtesy of Dr. Hatem Kalantan, associate professor, Department of Ophthalmology, King Saud University, Riyadh, SA).

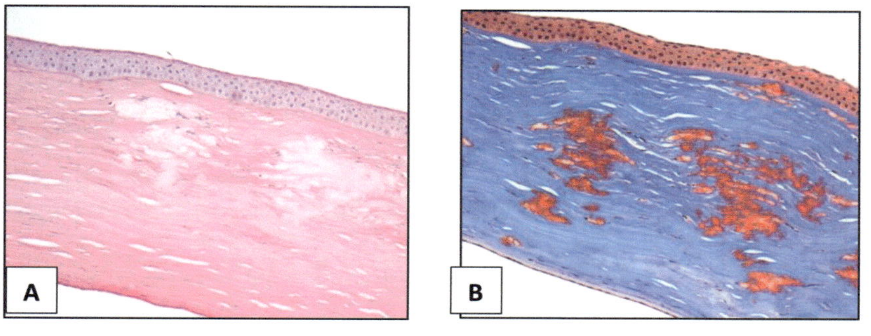

Figure 5.
(A) The histopathological appearance of the hyaline deposits in granular dystrophy (original magnification 200× periodic acid-Schiff) and (B) the same deposits highlighted using special stain (original magnification 200× Masson Trichrome).

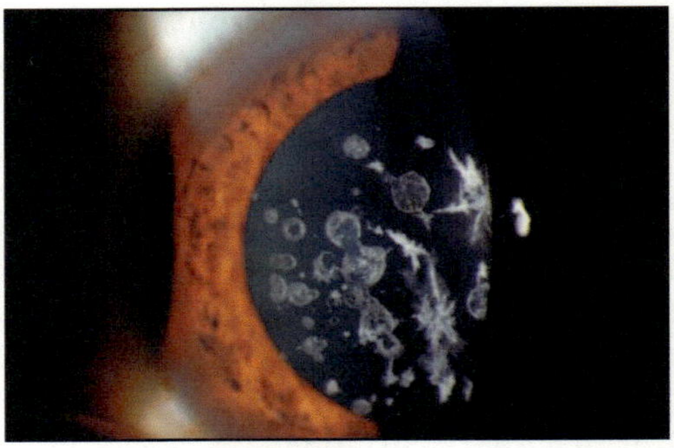

Figure 6.
The clinical appearance of Avellino dystrophy with classic combined spiky opacities as well as the granular deposits (courtesy of Dr. Majed Alkharashi, FRCS C, assistant professor, Department of Ophthalmology, King Saud University, Riyadh, SA).

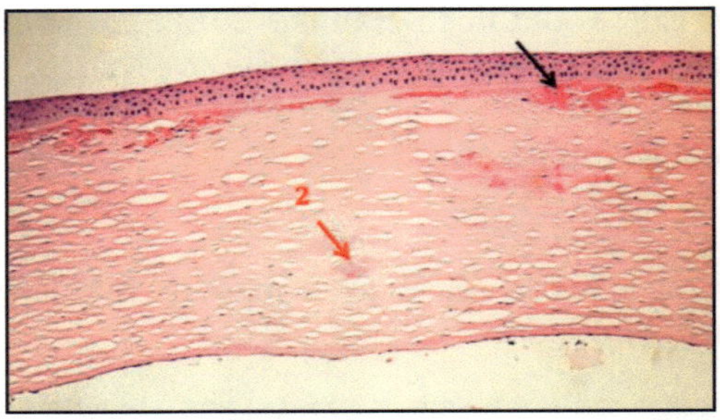

Figure 7.
The histopathological appearance of the two kinds of deposits: superficial hyaline deposits (black arrow) and the amyloid deposits (labeled as #2 with red arrow) deeper in the stroma (original magnification 100× periodic acid-Schiff).

Symptoms: recurrent erosive attacks. Visual deterioration occurs when visual axis is involved. Homozygotes are having a more rapid course.

Signs: initially, very small superficial stromal tiny whitish dots with small spokes that are usually arranged linearly like a string of pearls. With time, the center of the opacity fades resembling a ring. The anterior stromal deposits take the shape of spiky stars, icicles, or spider. The posterior corneal stroma may demonstrate linear or dot-like branching stromal opacities. The lines or dashes in GCD2 can be differentiated from LCD in that in GCD2 the lines are whiter, compared to the refractile nature of lattice lines in LCD. In addition, in GCD2, typically, the lines do not cross, while lattice lines in LCD characteristically intersect resulting in the lattice configuration. Compared to GCD1, patients with GCD2 have fewer stromal opacities (**Figure 6**). Homozygote patients present earlier with frequent superficial small dots and larger, dense superficial opacities in stroma that become deeper with age.

Histopathology: the abnormal corneal deposits extend from the basal epithelium to the deep stroma. Hyaline and amyloid materials are deposited and stain with Masson trichrome and/or Congo red (**Figure 7**). More severe histopathological findings are seen in homozygotes [3].

Management: treatment is usually not required. Refractive surgery is contraindicated.

3.3 Stromal dystrophies

The included dystrophies are:

1. Macular corneal dystrophy (MCD)

2. Schnyder corneal dystrophy (SCD)

3. Congenital stromal corneal dystrophy (CSCD)

4. Fleck corneal dystrophy (FCD)

5. Posterior amorphous corneal dystrophy (PACD)

6. Central cloudy dystrophy of François (CCDF)

7. Pre-Descemet corneal dystrophy (PDCD)

3.3.1 Macular corneal dystrophy (MCD)

Nomenclature: macular corneal dystrophy (MCD) is also known as Groenouw corneal dystrophy type II and Fehr spotted dystrophy [45, 46].

Inheritance: autosomal recessive.

Variants: Three variants that are clinically indistinguishable but on the basis of immunoreactivity of specific sulfated epitopes of antigenic keratan sulfates (AgKS) in the cornea and the serum:

1. MCD type I: no AgKS reactivity in the cornea and in the serum.

2. MCD type IA: keratocytes demonstrate AgKS reactivity, but not the extracellular tissue. No AgKS in the serum.

3. MCD type II: all deposits react with AgKS. Serum has normal or low levels of AgKS.

Genetic locus and gene: 16q22, carbohydrate sulfotransferase 6 gene—CHST6.

Category: C1.

Onset: during the first decade of life.

Symptoms: slowly progressive visual deterioration which becomes severe during the second and third decades. Light sensitivity and recurrent epithelial erosions can rarely be seen. Corneal sensation is reduced.

Signs: early in the course of the disease, central superficial whitish fleck-like opacities develop. Compared to GCD, these opacities extend peripherally to the limbus and the deep stroma down to Descemet's membrane. The intervening corneal stroma develops a progressive and diffuse haze (**Figure 8**). The epithelium is typically intact and, thus, corneal epithelial erosions are rare. The corneal thickness is reduced. Later in the course of the disease, corneal guttata and, rarely, endothelial decompensation occur.

Histopathology: glycosaminoglycans (GAGs) accumulate intracellularly and in the extracellular space and are better demonstrated with Alcian blue stain (**Figure 9A** and **B**). Breaks in the Bowman layer are observed. Stromal thinning and an overlying epithelial hyperplasia. Descemet's membrane and endothelium are involved. Descemet's membrane thickening and guttata are seen infrequently [3, 41]. Ultrastructural imaging and three-dimensional imaging of corneas with MCD demonstrate a clear organization of proteoglycans around the collagen fibrils. The collagen fibril diameter is significantly smaller than those of the normal cornea [47].

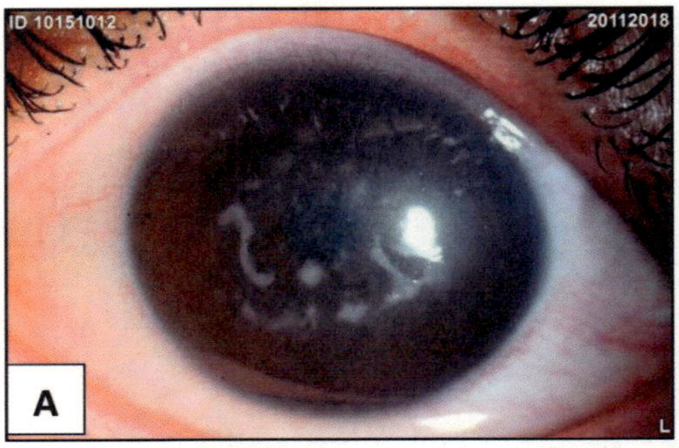

Figure 8.
The clinical appearance of macular dystrophy.

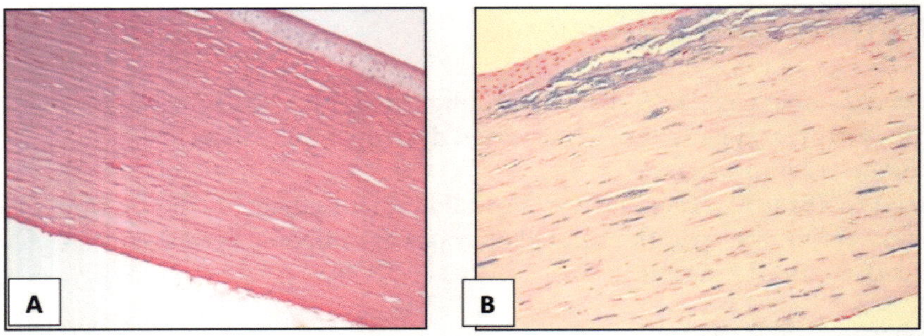

Figure 9.
(A) The histopathological appearance of the deposits in a case of macular dystrophy involving the full stromal thickness and the endothelium with secondary guttata (original magnification 200× periodic acid-Schiff) and (B) the glycosaminoglycan deposits in this dystrophy are demonstrated using Alcian blue stain (original magnification 200×).

Management: the treatment depends on the symptoms. Photophobia may be treated with lubrication and tinted contact lens. Superficial opacities can be treated with PTK and keratoplasty with deeper lesions. Recurrence may appear on the donor grafts [48].

3.3.2 Schnyder corneal dystrophy (SCD)

Inheritance: autosomal dominant.

Genetic locus and gene: 1p36, UbiA prenyltransferase domain containing 1—UBIAD1.

Category: C1.

Onset: the diagnosis is usually made during the second or third decade although onset may be in childhood. In patients with the crystalline form, diagnosis may be further delayed.

Symptoms: slowly progressive visual loss and glare. Scotopic vision is better than photopic vision. Corneal sensation decreases with age. It may be associated with hyperlipoproteinemia (type IIa, III, or IV). Significant visual deterioration usually occurs during the sixth decade.

Signs: clinical findings largely depend on the age of the patient. In patients who are 23 years or younger, a central round ring-like opacity or central comma-shaped subepithelial crystals are seen. Arcus lipoides usually develops in patients between 23 and 38 years of age. Diffuse stromal haze also develops after the age of 38. Almost 50% of patients demonstrate corneal crystals, which may be unilateral, and can occur late in the disease course.

Histopathology: intracellular and extracellular esterified and unesterified phospholipids and cholesterol are deposited in basal epithelial cells, Bowman's layer, and stroma. Fresh tissue stains positive with Oil Red O or Sudan black. Moreover, secondary amyloid and GAG depositions in cases with SCD were published [3].

Management: treatment is by excimer keratectomy or corneal transplantation procedures.

3.3.3 Congenital stromal corneal dystrophy (CSCD)

Inheritance: autosomal dominant.

Genetic locus and gene: 12q21.33, decorin, DCN.

Category: C1.

Onset: at birth.

Symptoms: variable degree of visual deterioration and less commonly photophobia. It is slowly progressive or even stationary.

Signs: diffuse, bilateral corneal clouding with whitish pan-stromal opacities. The corneal epithelium is intact. The corneal stroma is thicker than in normal individuals.

Histopathology: irregular separation of the corneal stromal lamellae that might contain amorphous material [3].

Management: spectacles or contact lenses for refractive errors, penetrating keratoplasty.

3.3.4 Fleck corneal dystrophy (FCD)

Inheritance: autosomal dominant.

Genetic locus and gene: 2q34, phosphoinositide kinase, FYVE finger containing— PIKFYVE.

Category: C1.

Onset: at birth or during the first years of life.

Symptoms: FCD is typically asymptomatic or associated with photophobia. It is a stationary dystrophy.

Signs: small, discrete, translucent, dandruff-like opacities scattered at any level of the corneal stroma and may extend to the limbus. The epithelium, Bowman's layer, Descemet's membrane, and endothelium are usually normal. The involvement can be asymmetric or unilateral.

Histopathology: the keratocytes are swollen and vacuolated and contain GAGs and complex lipids [3].

Management: treatment is usually not required.

3.3.5 Posterior amorphous corneal dystrophy (PACD)

Inheritance: autosomal dominant.

Genetic locus and gene: 12q21.33, deletion of keratocan (KERA), lumican (LUM), decorin (DCN), and epiphycan (EPYC).

Category: C1.

Onset: it is usually in the first decade of life.

Symptoms: mild slowly progressive, or nonprogressive, reduction of visual acuity.

Signs: diffuse gray sheet-like stromal opacities most prominent posteriorly. Corneal thinning is noted. Characteristic corneal flattening to less than 41 diopters with hyperopia. Descemet's membrane may be indented by the opacities.

Endothelial abnormalities have been reported. Other ocular associations include prominent Schwalbe's line, fine iris processes, pupillary remnants, iridocorneal adhesions, and iris hypoplasia. Notably, there is no associated glaucoma.

Histopathology: irregular posterior stromal lamellae. Positive staining with colloidal iron anterior to the Descemet's membrane. Localized attenuation of endothelial cells [3].

Management: if visual impairment is significant, penetrating keratoplasty is indicated.

3.3.6 Central cloudy dystrophy of Francois

Inheritance: mostly unknown. Autosomal dominant inheritance has been reported.

Genetic locus and gene: none.

Category: C4.

Onset: it usually presents in the first decade of life.

Symptoms: typically, asymptomatic.

Signs: nonprogressive central cloudy or rounded stromal opacities that are surrounded by clear tissue. It is clinically indistinguishable from posterior crocodile shagreen, a corneal degeneration. It has been associated with pseudoxanthoma elasticum, pre-Descemet's dystrophy, glaucoma, polymorphic amyloid degeneration, and keratoglobus.

Histopathology: no description has been reported in familial cases. Positive staining for GAGs [3].

Management: if visual impairment is significant, penetrating keratoplasty is indicated.

3.3.7 Pre-Descemet corneal dystrophy (PDCD)

Inheritance: there is no clear pattern of inheritance. It can be isolated although it has been described in certain families up to four generations. Autosomal dominant in inheritance in 1 pedigree has been reported in the punctiform and polychromatic PDCD. Deep corneal stromal opacities are frequently seen in X-linked ichthyosis.

Genetic locus and gene: isolated PDCD—unknown genetic locus and gene. PDCD associated with X-linked ichthyosis—Xp22.31, steroid sulfatase (STS).

Category: C1 in PDCD associated with X-linked ichthyosis. C4 in isolated PDCD.

Onset: usually during the fourth. However, it has been reported in children as young as 3 years.

Symptoms: typically, asymptomatic. Punctiform and polychromatic PDCD are stationary. Other forms are progressive.

Signs: the specific signs depend on the PDCD subgroups. Notably, many of the subgroups may represent sporadic or age-related degenerative changes. Deep stromal focal, fine opacities that may be central, annular, or diffuse. The changes are more uniform and polychromatic in an otherwise normal cornea in the punctiform and polychromatic subtypes.

Histopathology: enlarged keratocytes in the posterior corneal stroma containing vacuoles and intracytoplasmic inclusions of lipid-like material [3].

Management: usually not required.

3.4 Endothelial dystrophies

The included dystrophies are:

1. Fuchs endothelial corneal dystrophy (FECD)

2. Posterior polymorphous corneal dystrophy (PPCD)

3. Congenital hereditary endothelial dystrophy (CHED)

4. X-linked endothelial corneal dystrophy (XECD)

3.4.1 Fuchs endothelial corneal dystrophy (FECD)

FECD was first described in 1910 [49]. It is a noninflammatory, slowly progressive degeneration of endothelial cells which leads to corneal decompensation edema.

Inheritance: the genetic basis of FECD is complex and heterogeneous. Most cases are without a known inheritance pattern. Some autosomal dominant cases were reported.

Genetic locus and gene:

1. Early-onset FECD: 1p34.3-p32 (FECD1), collagen type VIII, alpha-2, COL8A2.

2. Late-onset FECD: reported genetic loci include 13pter-q12.13 (FECD2), 18q21.2-q21.3 (FECD3), 20p13-p12 (FECD4), 5q33.1-q35.2 (FECD5), 10p11.2 (FECD6), 9p24.1-p22.1 (FECD7), and 15q25 (FECD8). The gene is not identified.

Category: C1 in early-onset FECD, C2 in patients with identified genetic loci, and C3 in patients without known inheritance.

Onset: the patients are usually in the fourth decade or older. Early-onset FECD starts in the first decade. There is a female predominance at a ratio of 2.5:1 to 3:1.

Symptoms: progressive intermittent reduction in vision worse in the morning from epithelial/stromal edema caused by overnight eye closure. Epithelial erosions resulting from ruptured epithelial bullae typically cause pain, photophobia, and tearing. Patients also complain of progressive visual deterioration.

Signs: the signs of FECD can be reflected in four stages:

Stage 1: central cornea guttata that spreads peripherally. Some never progress to later stages. Corneal guttae in late-onset FECD are larger than those seen in early-onset FECD.

Stage 2: endothelial decompensation and stromal edema. Corneal endothelium has a beaten metal-like appearance with a thickened Descemet's membrane.

Stage 3: intraepithelial and interepithelial edema with epithelial bullae (bullous keratopathy).

Stage 4: subepithelial fibrosis, scarring, and peripheral superficial vascularization occurring in long-standing cases.

Histopathology: thickening and multilaminar Descemet's membrane with hyaline excrescences and atrophic endothelial cells that are reduced in number (**Figure 10**). There is an increasing waviness of the stromal collagen lamellae [3].

Management: treatment in early stages can be done by conservative measure. Hypertonic sodium chloride drops or ointment can be helpful [50]. Bandage contact lenses may alleviate pain from ruptured epithelial bullae. In advance cases a Descemet stripping endothelial keratoplasty (DSEK) procedure might be required either combined with cataract extraction or alone. In cases where there is opacification of the stroma, a full penetrating keratoplasty might be necessary [51].

3.4.2 Posterior polymorphous corneal dystrophy (PPCD)

Inheritance: autosomal dominant. Isolated nonhereditary unilateral cases have been reported.

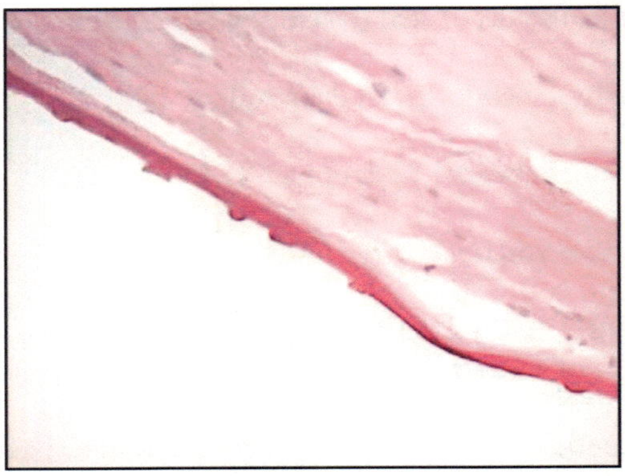

Figure 10.
Descemet's membrane appearance in a case of Fuchs' endothelial dystrophy with typical excrescences (original magnification 400× periodic acid-Schiff).

Genetic locus and gene: there are three known loci as follows:
PPCD 1: 20p11.2-q11.2, unknown gene
PPCD 2: 1p34.3-p32.3, collagen, type VIII, alpha-2 (COL8A2)
PPCD 3: 10p11.22, zinc finger E box–binding homeobox 1 (ZEB1)
Category: C2 in PPCD 1, C1 in PPCD 2 and PPCD 3.
Onset: during the first decade of life.

Symptoms: initially asymptomatic. Gradual visual loss occurs secondary to corneal edema. Endothelial changes often are possibly slowly progressive over years. Those changes may eventually lead to corneal decompensation.

Signs: asymmetric geographic gray opacities, vesicular lesions that can be single or grouped, usually in the inferior paracentral cornea. Gray-white endothelial bands with white flaky material along the bands. Diffuse opacification of Descemet's membrane and large vesicular endothelial opacities are seen in some cases. Guttata can be rarely seen. Corneal steepening has been reported, especially in PPCD 3, with corneal keratometry power of more than 48.0 diopters. Visually significant corneal edema, peripheral iridocorneal adhesions, and glaucoma are well-documented manifestations of PPCD.

Histopathology: focal fusiform or nodular excrescences formed by multiple layers of collagen on the posterior surface of Descemet's membrane. In addition, reduplication of the endothelial cell layer, blebs, or discontinuities is observed [3].

Management: treatment in the majority of patients is not indicated unless the patient is symptomatic; then treatment steps are similar to that of Fuchs endothelial corneal dystrophy.

3.4.3 Congenital hereditary endothelial dystrophy (CHED)

Inheritance: autosomal recessive.

Genetic locus and gene: 20p13, solute carrier family 4, sodium borate transporter, member 11—(SLC4A11) gene mutations.

Category: C1, C3 in cases without SLC4A11 mutations.

Onset: at birth.

Symptoms: nonprogressive congenital corneal clouding associated with blurred vision and nystagmus. Usually no tearing or photophobia.

Signs: bilateral variable limbus-to-limbus corneal clouding with occasional focal gray spots. Extensive corneal thickening (double or triple the normal corneal thickness). Rarely, secondary band keratopathy and elevated intraocular pressure. Significantly lower than normal endothelial cell count.

Histopathology: diffuse epithelial and pan-stromal edema associated with defects in the Bowman's layer. Degenerative and atrophic endothelial cells and a thickened laminated Descemet's membrane (**Figure 11**) [3]. Subepithelial amyloid deposition was found in 6.6% (**Figure 12**) [52].

Management: most CHED patients require corneal transplantation for visual rehabilitation. Better outcomes were seen with patients with delayed onset of the disease. Descemet stripping endothelial keratoplasty (DSEK) is an alternative to full-thickness keratoplasty for CHED with promising results [53–55].

3.4.4 X-linked endothelial corneal dystrophy (XECD)

Inheritance: X-chromosomal dominant.

Genetic locus and gene: Xq25, unknown gene.

Category: C2.

Onset: at birth.

Symptoms: asymptomatic and nonprogressive in females, minimally progressive decrease in vision in males.

Signs: in males, congenital corneal clouding that can range from diffuse haze to ground-glass and milky appearance of the cornea with possible nystagmus. It can present only with moon crater-like endothelial changes with or without secondary band keratopathy. In females, moon crater-like endothelial changes are observed.

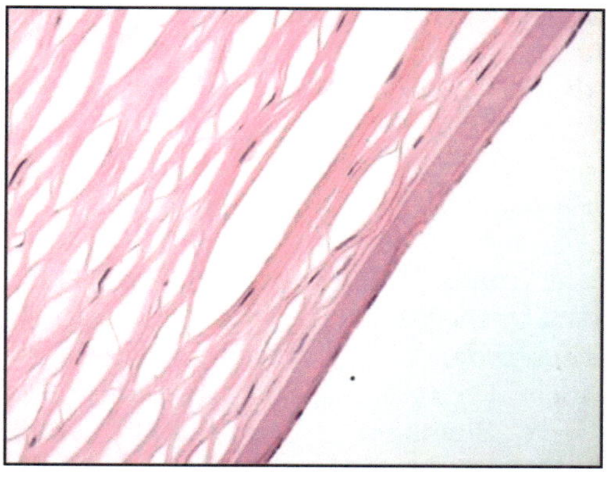

Figure 11.
The appearance of thick Descemet's membrane with attenuated endothelium in CHED (original magnification 400× periodic acid-Schiff).

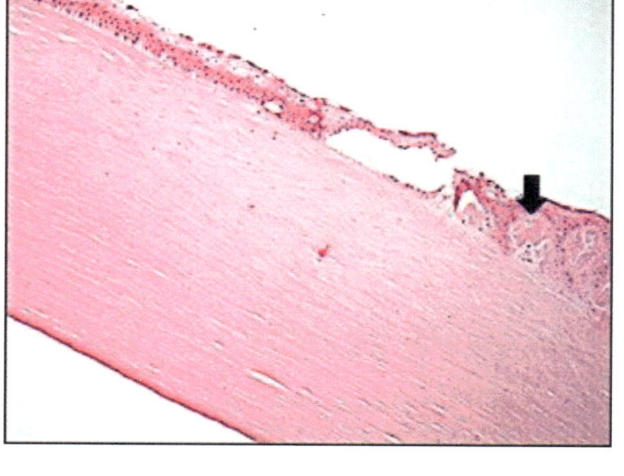

Figure 12.
Subepithelial amyloid deposits (black arrow head) in another case of CHED (original magnification 100× hematoxylin & eosin).

Histopathology: irregularity and thinning of the epithelium and Bowman's layer. Moon crater-like endothelial changes and subepithelial keratopathy. Irregularly arranged stromal collagen lamellae. Irregular thickening of Descemet's membrane with atypically appearance or loss of endothelial cells [3].

Management: a penetrating keratoplasty may be indicated in males in which corneal opacification significantly impairs vision.

4. Corneal degenerations

Corneal degenerations represent physiological decomposition or alteration of tissue elements and/or functions. They usually occur later in life with variable rate of progression and can be asymmetrical.

4.1 Epithelial and subepithelial degenerations

4.1.1 Pterygium

It is similar to pinguecula histopathologically where the substantia propria shows pseudo-elastotic changes, numerous blood vessels, and curly fibers but invades the cornea resulting in loss of Bowman's layer and epithelial changes (**Figure 13A** and **B**). They can cause astigmatism, interfere with contact lens fitting, and may cause ocular motility restriction. Advanced pterygia are treated surgically with the use of antimetabolites or conjunctival graft [56].

4.1.2 Environmental proteinaceous corneal degeneration (EPCD)

Previously known as "spheroidal degeneration" or "climatic droplet keratopathy." It is characterized by the presence of yellowish aggregates that accumulate near the limbus and then progressively extend toward the central part of the cornea within the palpebral fissure. The globular amorphous material is primarily deposited in the area of Bowman's layer and can be demonstrated using an elastic stain (**Figure 14**). It can be primary or secondary, affecting males, and is related to cornea microtrauma caused by wind, dust, and ultraviolet radiation [57, 58].

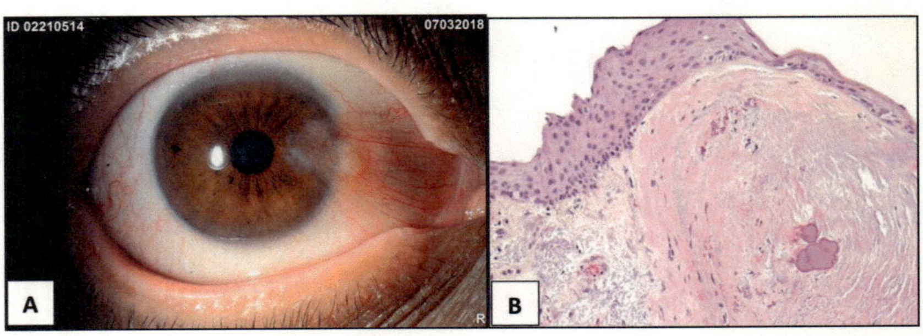

Figure 13.
(A) The clinical appearance of a nasal pterygium and (B) pterygium showing pseudo-elastotic degeneration with an area of limbal stroma and climatic droplet keratopathy (CDK) deposits (original magnification 200× hematoxylin & eosin).

4.2 Stromal (central)

Central stromal degenerations include:

1. Mosaic (crocodile) shagreen

2. Cornea farinata

3. Polymorphic amyloid degeneration

4.3 Peripheral stromal

Peripheral stromal degenerations include:

1. White limbal girdle of Vogt: types I and II

2. Corneal arcus

3. Senile furrow degeneration

4. Terrien's marginal degeneration

4.4 Post-inflammatory corneal degenerations

4.4.1 Band-shaped keratopathy

Occurs as dense calcium deposits in the form of whitish calcium hydroxyapatite or yellowish hydroxyl apatite and phosphate within the superficial cornea and Bowman's layer across the interpalpebral fissure (**Figure 15**). Common causes include hypercalcemia of variable etiology, chronic ocular diseases such as uveitis, and gout, and it can be idiopathic. It can be safely treated by calcium chelation using warm neutral disodium ethylenediaminetetraacetic acid (EDTA) [59].

4.4.2 Salzmann's nodular degeneration

Initially described in 1925 as a nodular post-inflammatory keratopathy resulting in disruption of Bowman's layer, subepithelial fibrosis and vascularization [60].

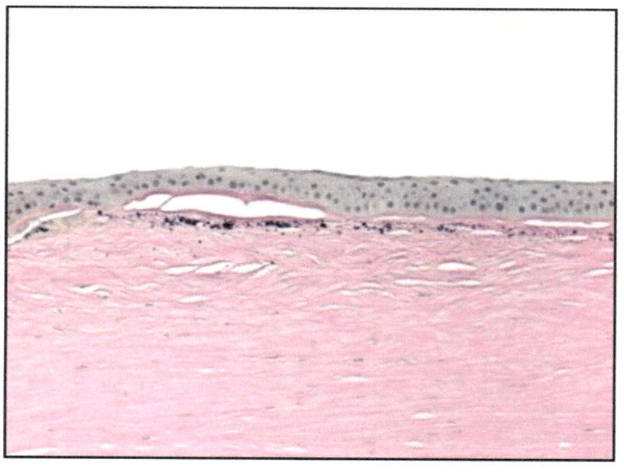

Figure 14.
An early case of CDK with the deposits at Bowman's layer level (original magnification 200× elastic stain).

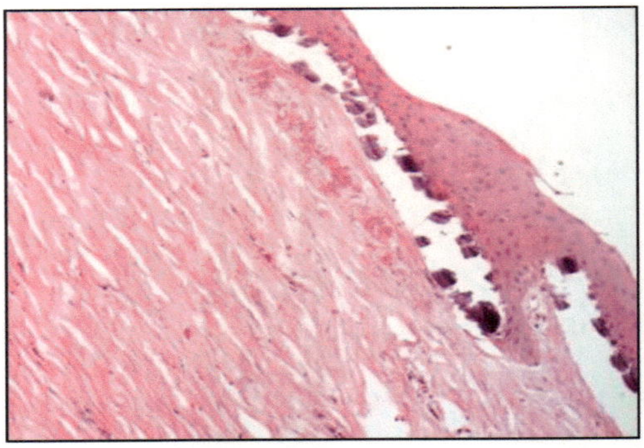

Figure 15.
The corresponding subepithelial calcium deposits (original magnification 400× hematoxylin & eosin).

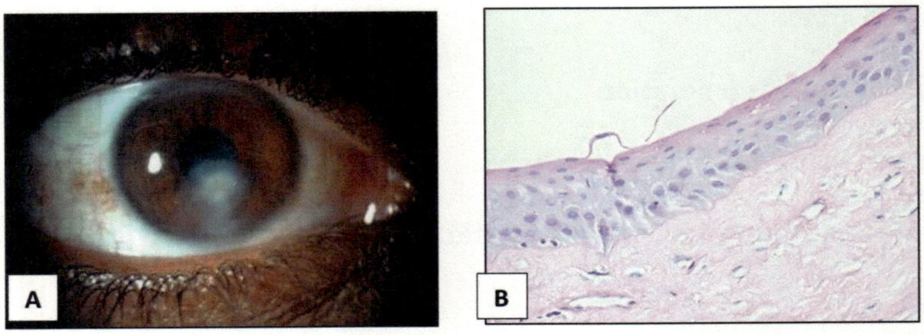

Figure 16.
(A) Clinical case of peripheral hypertrophic subepithelial corneal degeneration (PHSD) and (B) epithelial thickening, absence of Bowman's layer and subepithelial fibrosis in a similar case of PHSD (original magnification X400 periodic acid-Schiff).

It appears to affect middle-aged women and to have good prognosis if properly treated medically using lubrication and surgically by superficial keratectomy [61].

The electron microscopy of these nodules shows irregular lamellae, and keratocytes that are covered by an interrupted basement membrane Bowman's layer is replaced by collagenous material, which shows positive vimentin straining [57].

4.4.3 Peripheral hypertrophic subepithelial corneal degeneration

It is a more recently recognized uncommon corneal degeneration, which is typically peri-limbal, slowly progressive, and bilateral. It tends to occur in white women with unknown etiology and, however, resembles Salzmann's nodular degeneration in appearance (**Figure 16A** and **B**) [62, 63]. Ultraviolet radiation and limbal insufficiency have been proposed in the pathogenesis [64].

The fibrotic process has been linked to low-grade inflammation with low TGF F-B1 concentrations [62]. Surgical excision might be required for treatment of symptomatic cases, and the recurrence is not common [63].

4.4.4 Others

Amyloid degeneration and lipid keratopathy.

4.5 Endothelial

Hassall-Henle bodies.

4.6 Corneal pigmentations

Iron lines: there are multiple theories behind the formation of such lines with iron deposits typically within the corneal epithelium at various levels [57]. They include:

1. Hudson-Stahli line: in aging cornea

2. Stocker's line: at the edge of chronic pterygium

3. Fleischer's ring: at the base of the corneal protruding cone in keratoconus

4. Ferry's line: in front of a filtering bleb

5. Ectatic corneal disorders

5.1 Keratoconus

Dudell in 1729 described a patient with protruding cornea and deteriorating vision; this was the earliest references to keratoconus [65]. Initial classification of the disease was dependent on the clinical pattern of the ectatic cone and included round or nipple cones with a central or oval protrusion and oval cones (**Figure 17A**). Amsler contributed to the disease detection by using a Placido's disk to determine early cases [66]. In the 1980s, the first color-coded Placido map of corneal curvature was published and led to multiple commercially available computerized video-keratoscopes [67, 68]. Then the more detailed elevation-based topographic devices and pachymetric mapping were developed and enabled more through assessment of the condition.

The onset of keratoconus typically begins at puberty but might begin during childhood and undergoes variable progression until the third or fourth decade [69–71]. It is a bilateral condition that is highly asymmetrical that can be associated with atopy, Down's syndrome, Leber's congenital amaurosis, retinitis pigmentosa, Marfan's syndrome, and mitral valve prolapse [65, 72].

It can present as a sporadic condition; a positive family history has been documented not infrequently. It is suggested that that there is an autosomal dominant form of the disorder with variable phenotypic expression in 90% of those with familial keratoconus [65, 73].

The symptoms may vary widely depending on the degree of astigmatism, degree of irregularity, and presence of scarring. Slit lamp findings may include the presence of a Fleischer's ring, which is iron epithelial deposits (described earlier), and can be

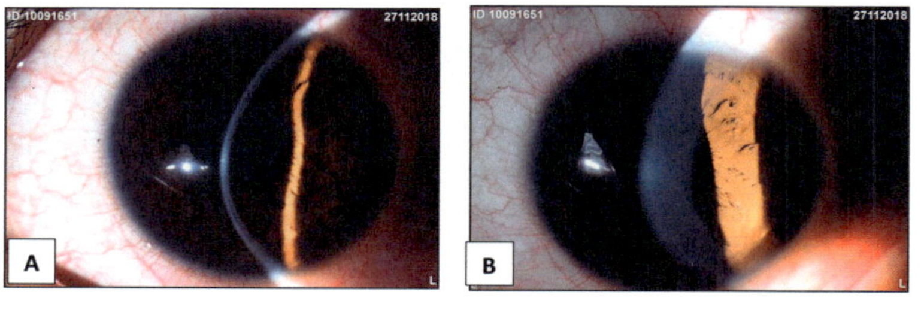

Figure 17.
(A) The clinical thinning of the ectatic cornea in keratoconus (KC) and (B) a Fleischer ring indicating iron deposition around the cone in a case of keratoconus.

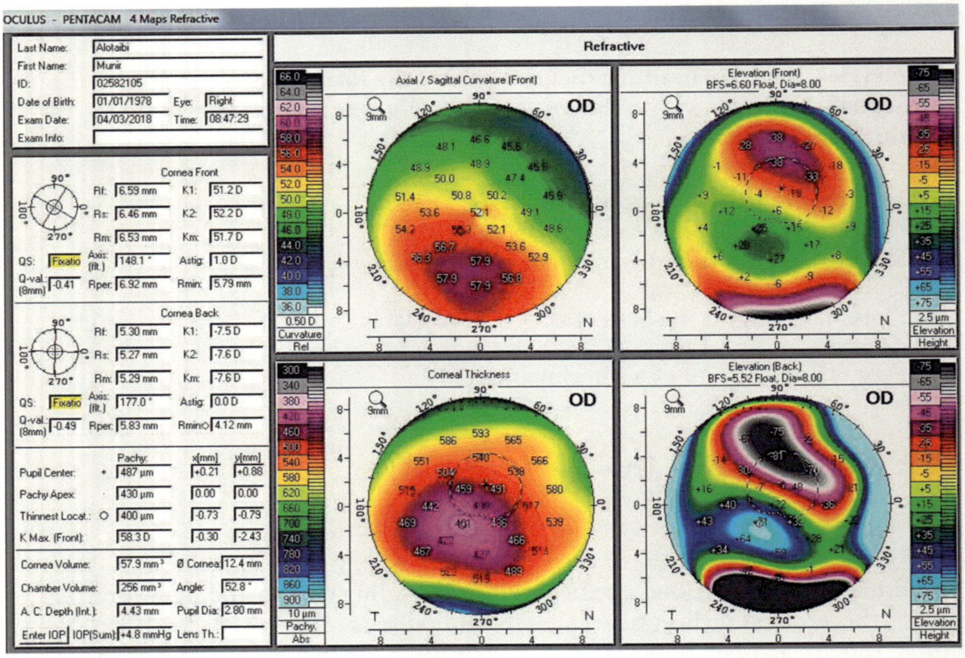

Figure 18.
Topography showing steep keratometry maps with irregular astigmatism mirroring the area of thinning with high reading on anterior and posterior elevation maps.

seen better with the use of the cobalt blue filter (**Figure 17B**) [72]. Reticular scarring at the level of bowman's lay can be seen as well as striations in Descemet's membrane and the deep stroma (Vogt's striae). These striations represent corneal stress lines that parallel the axis of the cone [65, 74]. In advanced cases of keratoconus, Munson's sign and Rizzuti's sign can also be seen on gross inspection [75]. Ophthalmoscopy can show the outline of the early cone as an oil droplet against the background red reflex of the fundus. Retinoscopy on a patient with early keratoconus may show scissoring of the retinoscopic reflex. In cases of severe keratoconus, individuals might develop an acute onset of pain, blurred vision, and photophobia. Examination reveals diffuse corneal edema that results from a break in Descemet's membrane.

The ability to detect early and subclinical (forme fruste) keratoconus might be difficult depending on clinical examination alone. The use of corneal topographies has improved our ability to distinguish very early cases. Many indices were proposed and artificial intelligence methods such as the KISA% index and the Rabinowitz-McDonnell test have all been developed to help diagnose keratoconus in different stages of the disease and most importantly in early cases. Recent efforts looking at the relational thickness of the central and peripheral cornea have been helpful in the early detection of disease [76]. Modern elevation-based corneal topography provides three-dimensional reconstruction of the cornea enabling evaluation of the anterior and posterior corneal surfaces and assessing the thickness maps (**Figure 18**).

Histopathological studies of corneas with keratoconus demonstrated breaks in Bowman's layer or the complete absence of the layer, stromal collagen disorganization, scarring, and generalized central thinning of the stroma (**Figure 19A**).

Treatment options start with spectacle correction, toric soft contact lens, and hard contact lens wear. In some cases, the use of intrastromal corneal implants might be helpful. Keratoplasty (lamellar or penetrating) is reserved for more advanced cases with an overall good success rate (**Figure 19B**).

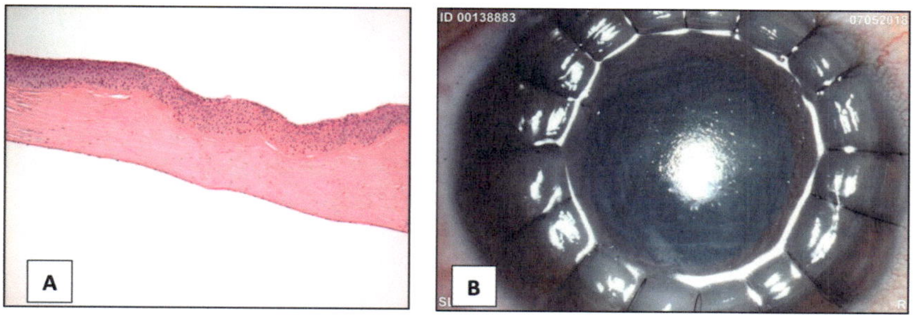

Figure 19.
(A) The evident stromal thinning with compensatory thickening of the epithelium and breaks in Bowman's layer in KC (original magnification 100× periodic acid-Schiff) and (B) the postoperative appearance of lamellar keratoplasty done for a patient with keratoconus.

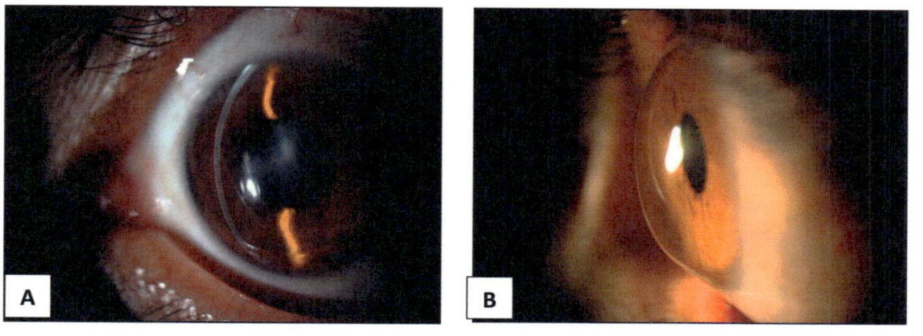

Figure 20.
(A) Slit lamp lit appearance of peripheral corneal thinning in a case of pellucid marginal degeneration (PMD) and (B) side view of the inferior corneal bulge in PMD.

5.2 Pellucid marginal degeneration

Pellucid marginal degeneration (PMD) is an ectatic corneal disease that is progressive, bilateral noninflammatory, with thinning involving the inferior cornea in a crescentic pattern [65]. Typically, this thinning occurs inferiorly 1–3 mm from the limbus (**Figure 20A** and **B**). A band of normal cornea is found inferior to the ectatic area. This configuration causes the superior cornea to protrude over the ectasia causing a "beer belly" configuration [77]. PMD affecting the superior cornea is documented in the literature [78–81]. There might be an association with vernal keratoconjunctivitis, atopy, and frequent rubbing of the ocular surface [65].

It can be managed by hard contact lenses or soft toric contact lens. Surgical treatment options are technically difficult and have lower success rates than in keratoconus. Crescentic lamellar keratoplasty, epikeratoplasty, and corneal wedge/resection all have been attempted with variable results.

5.3 Keratoglobus

Keratoglobus is a rare, noninflammatory ectatic disorder characterized by bilateral corneal from limbus to limbus. The corneal diameter is typically normal, and the cornea is clear, except in cases of hydrops. It can be associated with two autosomal recessive diseases, Ehlers-Danlos and Blue-Sclera syndrome. Acquired keratoglobus may appear de novo or may be associated with other ocular diseases, such as vernal keratoconjunctivitis, blepharitis, Leber's congenital amaurosis, and thyroid ophthalmopathy [82].

Penetrating keratoplasty, while the classical surgical treatment for other corneal diseases, is not appropriate in keratoglobus patients. Other procedures, such as inlay lamellar keratoplasty and limbus-to-limbus epikeratoplasty, have been attempted with variable results [83–85]. Preferably a spectacle correction as this also provides protection from rupture. Contact lenses can also be used.

Conflict of interest

We do not have any financial interests in any of the listed items in this manuscript.

Author details

Hind Alkatan*, Norah Alkheraiji and Tariq Alzahem
King Saud University, Riyadh, Kingdom of Saudi Arabia

*Address all correspondence to: hindkatan@yahoo.com

References

[1] Kanski JJ, Bowling B, Nischal KK, Pearson A. Cornea. Clinical Ophthalmology: A Systematic Approach. 8th ed. Edinburgh, New York: Elsevier/Saunders; 2016. pp. 168-237

[2] AAo O. Basic and Clinical Science Course Section 8: External Disease and Cornea. San Francisco, CA: American Academy of Ophthalmology; 2015. pp. 253-287

[3] Weiss JS, Moller HU, Aldave AJ, Seitz B, Bredrup C, Kivela T, et al. IC3D classification of corneal dystrophies—Edition 2. Cornea. 2015;**34**(2):117-159

[4] Friedlaender MH, Smolin G. Corneal degenerations. Annals of Ophthalmology. 1979;**11**(10):1485-1495

[5] Sacca SC, Roszkowska AM, Izzotti A. Environmental light and endogenous antioxidants as the main determinants of non-cancer ocular diseases. Mutation Research. 2013;**752**(2):153-171

[6] Harayama K, Amemiya T, Nishimura H. Development of the cornea during fetal life: Comparison of corneal and bulbar diameter. The Anatomical Record. 1980;**198**(3):531-535

[7] Graw J. Eye development. Current Topics in Developmental Biology. 2010;**90**:343-386

[8] Robert A Copeland J, Afshari NA, Dohlman CH. Corneal Embryology, Copeland and Afshari's Principles and Practice of Cornea. Vol. 1. New Delhi; London: Jaypee Brothers Medical Publishers; 2013. pp. 16-25

[9] Ehlers N, Hjortdal J. The biology of the eye. 1st ed. Bittar EE, editor. Amsterdam: Elsevier; 2006. 87 p.

[10] Hay ED. Development of the vertebrate cornea. International Review of Cytology. 1980;**63**:263-322

[11] Bannister LH, Berry MM, Collins P, et al. Gray's Anatomy. 38th ed. Edinburgh: Churchill Livingstone; 1999. 259 p

[12] Moore KL, Persaud TVN, Shiota K. Color Atlas of Clinical Embryology. Philadelphia: WB Saunders; 1994

[13] Harayama K, Amemiya T, Nishimura H. Development of the eyeball during fetal life. Journal of Pediatric Ophthalmology and Strabismus. 1981;**18**(4):37-40

[14] Trevor-Roper PD. The eye and its disorders. 1. The eyeball. International Ophthalmology Clinics. 1974;**14**(1-2):3-25

[15] Styszyński A, Bruska M, Woźniak W. Morphometric study of the cornea in human embryos. Morphometric study of the cornea in human embryos. Folia Morphologica. 2001;**60**(1):57-59

[16] Wulle KG, Richter J. Electron microscopy of the early embryonic development of the human corneal epithelium. Albrecht von Graefes Archiv fur klinische und experimentelle Ophthalmologie—Albrecht von Graefe's Archive for Clinical and Experimental Ophthalmology. 1978;**209**(1):39-49

[17] Sowden JC. Molecular and developmental mechanisms of anterior segment dysgenesis. Eye (London, England). 2007;**21**(10):1310-1318

[18] Copeland Jr RA, Afshari NA, Dohlman CH. Basic Structure and Function of the Human Cornea and Adnexal Structures, Corneal Embryology, Copeland and Afshari's Principles and Practice of Cornea. Vol. 1. New Delhi; London: Jaypee Brothers Medical Publishers; 2013. pp. 3-18

[19] AAo O. Basic and Clinical Science Course. Section 2: Fundamentals and Principles of Ophthalmology. San

Francisco, CA: American Academy of Ophthalmology; 2014. pp. 44-45

[20] Ophthalmology AAo. Basic and Clinical Science Course Section 8: External Disease and Cornea. San Francisco, CA: American Academy of Ophthalmology; 2014. p. 74

[21] Ophthalmology AAo. Basic and Clinical Science Course. Section 8: External Disease and Cornea. San Francisco, CA: American Academy of Ophthalmology; 2014. p. 9

[22] Dua HS, Faraj LA, Said DG, Gray T, Lowe J. Human corneal anatomy redefined: A novel pre-Descemet's layer (Dua's layer). Ophthalmology. 2013;**120**:1778-1785

[23] The IC3D Classification of the Corneal Dystrophies. Cornea. 2008;**27**:S1-S42

[24] Cogan DG, Donaldson DD, Kuwabara T, et al. Microcystic dystrophy of the corneal epithelium. Transactions of the American Ophthalmological Society. 1964;**62**:213-225

[25] Laibson PR, Krachmer JH. Familial occurrence of dot, map, fingerprint dystrophy of the cornea. Investigative Ophthalmology & Visual Science. 1975;**14**:397-399

[26] Werblin TP, Hirst LW, Stark WJ, et al. Prevalence of map-dot-fingerprint changes in the cornea. The British Journal of Ophthalmology. 1981;**65**:401-409

[27] Boutboul S, Black GCM, Moore JE, et al. A subset of patients with epithelial basement membrane corneal dystrophy have mutations in TGFBI/BIGH3. Human Mutation. 2006;**27**:553-557

[28] Meesmann A, Wilke F. Klinische und anatomische Untersuchungen uber eine bisher unbekannte, dominant vererbte Epithel Dystrophie der Horn haut. Klinische Monatsblätter für Augenheilkunde, Stuttgart. 1939;**103**:361-391

[29] Burns RP. Meesmann's corneal dystrophy. Transactions of the American Ophthalmological Society. 1968;**66**:530-635

[30] Chiou AG, Florakis GJ, Copeland RL, et al. Recurrent Meesmann's corneal epithelial dystrophy after penetrating keratoplasty. Cornea. 1998;**17**:566-570

[31] Lisch W, Steuhl KP, Lisch C, et al. A new, band-shaped and whorled microcystic dystrophy of the corneal epithelium. American Journal of Ophthalmology. 1992;**114**:35-44

[32] Wessel MM, Sarkar J, Jakobiec FA, et al. Treatment of Lisch corneal dystrophy with photorefractive keratectomy and Mitomycin C. Cornea. 2011;**30**:481-485

[33] Nakaizumi GA. A rare case of corneal dystrophy. Acta Societatis Ophthalmologicae Japonicae. 1914;**18**:949-950

[34] Zhang B, Yao YF. Gelatinous drop-like corneal dystrophy with a novel mutation of TACSTD2 manifested in combination with spheroidal degeneration in a Chinese patient. Molecular Vision. 2010;**16**:1570-1575

[35] Reis W. Familiare, fleckige Hornhautentartung. Deutsche Medizinische Wochenschrift. 1917;**43**:575

[36] Thiel HJ, Behnke H. Eine bisher unbekannte subepitheliale hereditare Hornhautdystophie. Klinische Monatsblätter für Augenheilkunde. 1967;**150**:862-874

[37] Gear HC, Ramaesh K, Roberts F. Recurrence of Thiel-Behnke corneal dystrophy: An electron microscopic

study. The British Journal of Ophthalmology. 2005;**89**:518-520

[38] Wittebol-Post D, Van Schooneveld MJ. The corneal dystrophy of Waardenburg and Jonkers. Ophthalmic Paediatrics and Genetics. 1989;**10**:249-255

[39] Ridgway AE, Akhtar S, Munier FL, et al. Ultrastructural and molecular anaylysis of Bowman's layer corneal dystrophies: An epithelial origin? Investigative Ophthalmology & Visual Science. 2000;**41**:3286-3292

[40] Seitz B, Behrens A, Fischer M, et al. Morphometric analysis of deposits in granular and lattice corneal dystrophy: Histopathologic implications for phototherapeutic keratectomy. Cornea. 2004;**23**(4):380-385

[41] Alzuhairy S, Alkatan HM, Al-Rajhi AA. Prevalence and histopathological characteristics of corneal stromal dystrophies in Saudi Arabia. Middle East African Journal of Ophthalmology. 2015;**22**(2):179-185

[42] Yao YF, Jin YQ, Zhang B, et al. Recurrence of lattice corneal dystrophy caused by incomplete removal of stroma after deep lamellar keratoplasty. Cornea. 2006;**25**(10 Suppl. 1):S41-S46

[43] Meyer HJ. Prognosis of keratoplasty in hereditary stromal dystrophies. Klinische Monatsblätter für Augenheilkunde. 1996;**208**(6):446-449

[44] Lyons CJ, McCartney AC, Kirkness CM. Granular corneal dystrophy. Visual results and pattern of recurrence after lamellar or penetrating keratoplasty. Ophthalmology. 1994;**101**(11):1812-1817

[45] Di Iorio E, Barbaro V, Volpi N, et al. Localization and expression of CHST6 and keratan sulfate proteoglycans in the human cornea. Experimental Eye Research. 2010;**91**(2):293-299

[46] Waring GO 3rd, Rodrigues MM, Laibson PR. Corneal dystrophies: Dystrophies of the epithelium, Bowman's layer and stroma. Survey of Ophthalmology. 1978;**23**(2):71-122

[47] Akhtar S, Alkatan HM, Kirat O, Khan AA, Almubrad T. Collagen fibrils and proteoglycans of macular dystrophy cornea: Ultrastructure and 3D transmission electron tomography. Microscopy and Microanalysis: The Official Journal of Microscopy Society of America, Microbeam Analysis Society, Microscopical Society of Canada. 2015;**21**(3):666-679

[48] Szentmary N, Seitz B, Langenbucher A, et al. Histologic and ultrastructural changes in corneas with granular and macular dystrophy after excimer laser phototherapeutic keratectomy. Cornea. 2006;**25**(3):257-263

[49] Fuchs E. Dystrophia epithelialis corneae. Graefe's Archive for Clinical and Experimental Ophthalmology. 1910;**76**:48-508

[50] Adamis AP, Filatov V, Tripathi BJ, et al. Fuchs' endothelial dystrophy of the cornea. Survey of Ophthalmology. 1993;**38**:149-168

[51] Price MO, Price DA, Fairchild KM, et al. Rate and risk factors for cataract formation and extraction after Descemet stripping endothelial keratoplasty. The British Journal of Ophthalmology. 2010;**94**:1468-1471

[52] Al-Shehah A, Al-Rajhi A, Alkatan H. Amyloid corneal deposition in corneal buttons of congenital hereditary endothelial dystrophy (CHED)—A clinical and histopathological case series. Saudi Journal of Ophthalmology: Official Journal of the Saudi Ophthalmological Society. 2010;**24**(4):111-118

[53] Sajjadi H, Javadi MA, Hemmati R, et al. Results of penetrating keratoplasty

in CHED. Congenital hereditary endothelial dystrophy. Cornea. 1995;**14**:18-25

[54] Busin M, Beltz J, Scorcia V. Descemet-stripping automated endothelial keratoplasty for congenital hereditary endothelial dystrophy. Archives of Ophthalmology. 2011;**129**:1140-1146

[55] Schmid E, Lisch W, Philipp W, et al. A new, X-linked endothelial corneal dystrophy. American Journal of Ophthalmology. 2006;**141**:478-487

[56] Kim KW, Kim JC. Current approaches and future directions in the management of pterygium. International Journal of Ophthalmology. 2018;**II**(5):709-711

[57] Tabarra KF, Alkatan HM. Climatic droplet keratopathy. In: Copeland and Afshari's Principles and Practice of Cornea, Chapter 46. India: Jaypee-Highlights Medical Publishers; 2013. pp. 559-566

[58] Serra HM, Suarez MF, Urrets-Zavalia JA. Environmental protenaceous corneal degeneration: A rare disease. In: Chapter 1 in Rare Disease. Available from: www.avidscience.com

[59] Al-Hilty A, Ramaesh K, Lockington D. EDTA chelation for symptomatic band Keratopathy: Results and recurrence. Eye (London, England). 2018;**32**(1):26-31. DOI: 10.1038/eye.2017.264

[60] Lanier JD. Salzmann's nodular degeneration (subepithelial fibrosis). Ophthalmic Surgery, Laser and Imaging. 2011;**42**(4):350-352

[61] Farjo AA, Halperin GI, Syed N, Sutphin JE, Wagoner MD. Salzmann's nodular corneal degeneration clinical characteristics and surgical outcomes. Cornea. 2006;**25**(1):11-15

[62] Jarventausta PJ, Tervo TMT, Kivela T, Holopainen JM. Peripheral hypertrophic subepithelial corneal degenerate clinical and histopathological features. Acta Ophthalmologica. 2014;**92**:774-782

[63] Gore DM, Iovieno A, Connel BJ, Alexander A, Meligonis G, Dart JK. Peripheral hypertrophic subepithelial corneal degeneration: Nomendature, phenotypes, and long-term outcomes. Ophthalmology. 2013;**120**:892-898

[64] Schargus M, Kusserow C, Schlotzer-Schrehanat U, Hofmann Rummelt C, Schlunk G, Geerlong G. Peripheral hypertrophic subepithelial corneal degeneration presenting with bilateral nasal and temporal corneal changes. Eye. 2015;**29**:88-97

[65] Krachmer JH, Feder RS, Belin MW. Keratoconus and related noninflammatory corneal thinning disorders. Survey of Ophthalmology. 1984;**28**:293-322

[66] Amsler M. Keraton classique et keratocone fruste, augments unitaires. Ophthalmologica. 1946;**11**:96-101

[67] Rabinowitz YS, McDonnell PJ. Computer-assisted corneal topography in keratoconus. Refractive & Corneal Surgery. 1989;**5**:400-408

[68] Maeda N, Klyce SD, Smolek MK, et al. Automated keratoconus screening with corneal topography analysis. Investigative Ophthalmology & Visual Science. 1994;**35**:2749-2757

[69] Wagner H, Barr JT, Zadnik K. Collaborative longitudinal evaluation of Keratoconus (CLEK) study: Methods and findings to date. Contact Lens & Anterior Eye. 2007;**30**:223-232

[70] Owens H, Gamble G. A profile of keratoconus in New Zealand. Cornea. 2003;**22**:122-125

[71] Crews MJ, Driebe WT, Stern GA. The clinical management of keratoconus: A

6 year retrospective study. The CLAO Journal. 1994;**20**:194-197

[72] Wilson SE, Klyce SD. Advances in the analysis of corneal topography. Survey of Ophthalmology. 1991;**35**:269-277

[73] Falls HF, Allen AW. Dominantly inherited keratoconus. Journal de Génétique Humaine. 1969;**17**:317-324

[74] Zadnik K, Barr JT, Gordon MO, et al. Biomicroscopic signsand disease severity in keratoconus. Collaborative longitudinal evaluation of Keratoconus (CLEK) study group. Cornea. 1996;**15**:139-146

[75] Ihalainen A. Clinical and epidemiological features of keratoconus genetic and external factors in the pathogenesis of the disease. Acta Ophthalmologica. Supplement. 1986;**178**:1-64

[76] Ambrosio R, Alonso RS, Luz A, et al. Corneal-thickness spatial profile and corneal-volume distribution: Tomographic indices to detect keratoconus. Journal of Cataract and Refractive Surgery. 2006;**32**:1851-1859

[77] Tzelikis PF, Cohen EJ, Rapuano CJ, et al. Management of pellucid marginal corneal degeneration. Cornea. 2005;**24**:555-560

[78] Wagenhorst BB. Unilateral pellucid marginal degeneration in an elderly patient. The British Journal of Ophthalmology. 1996;**80**:927-928

[79] Ertan A, Bahadir M. Management of superior pellucid marginal degeneration with a single intracorneal ring segment using femtosecond laser. Journal of Refractive Surgery. 2007;**23**:205-208

[80] Sridhar MS, Mahesh S, Bansal AK, et al. Superior pellucid marginal corneal degeneration. Eye. 2004;**18**:393-399

[81] Bower KS, Dhaliwal DK, Barnhorst DA, et al. Pellucid marginal degeneration with superior thinning. Cornea. 1997;**16**:483-485

[82] Gonzalez V, McDonnell PJ. Computer-assisted corneal topography in parents of patients with keratoconus. Archives of Ophthalmology. 1992;**110**:1413-1414

[83] Jones D, Kirkness C. A new surgical technique for keratoglobus—tectonic lamellar keratoplasty followed by secondary penetrating keratoplasty (case reports). Cornea. 2001;**20**:885-887

[84] Kanellopoulos J, Lawrence H. An alternative surgical procedure for the management of keratoglobus. Cornea. 2005;**24**:1024-1026

[85] Vajpayee R, Bhartiya P, Sharma N. Central lamellar keratoplasty with peripheral intralamellar tuck: A new surgical technique for keratoglobus. Cornea. 2002;**21**:657-660

Chapter 2

Optical Coherence Tomography in the Management of Glaucoma and Macular Diseases

Lawan Abdu

Abstract

Optical coherence tomography (OCT) is a non contact, non invasive and reproducible imaging technique that produces thin slices of tissue section images. OCT identifies retinal nerve fiber damage before detection of visual field changes making it a handy and effective tool in early detection and monitoring in glaucoma. Retinal fiber layer thickness measurements provide vital knowledge of extent of neural damage. This enables the clinician to counsel the patient and take the best decision towards achieving glaucoma control. Early and quantifiable macular thickness measurements are obtained, allowing for detection of clinically significant diabetic macular edema. OCT allows monitoring of the impact of laser or other interventions. Changes in age-related macular degeneration are relatively easily determined and impact of treatment interventions monitored. In conclusion, OCT is a vital emerging tool in the evaluation and management glaucoma and macular diseases in all parts of the World, including low income countries of sub-Saharan Africa.

Keywords: OCT, glaucoma, macular, diseases, management

1. Introduction

Optical coherence tomography (OCT) is a noninvasive, noncontact, and reproducible investigation. The relatively new technology is comparable to ultrasound that utilizes low coherence interferometry to produce cross-sectional images of the retina. The functional principle behind OCT imaging is light interference [1]. Infrared light from a luminescent diode source is divided into two, one of which is reflected from a reference mirror and the other scattered from retinal tissues. The reflected beams from the two sources are made to produce interference pattern, thus obtaining the echo time delay and their amplitude information which makes up an A-scan. The cross-sectional images are generated by measuring the echo time delay and intensity of light reflected from internal structures in the retina [2]. Scattering is a property of heterogonous medium and arises due to variation in refractive index between tissues structures. An interferometric technique analyzes the reflected light signal, and a transverse scanning mechanism captures the A-scans from adjoining retinal locations to produce a two-dimensional image [3]. OCT produces high-resolution images which allows detailed assessment of retinal thickness and morphologic evaluation of retinal layers [4]. The image is colored to enhance tissue recognition. There are two models described: time domain (TD-OCT) and Fourier domain (FD-OCT). In TD-OCT, measurements of the light echoes are detected sequentially by stepwise movement of the reference mirror, while in FD-OCT, the light echoes and the source from all axial depth are detected as modulations in the source spectrum simultaneously [5]. One of the main differences is the reference mirror in TD-OCT. The moving mirror causes inertia and limits mechanical performance of the TD-OCT. Elimination of this mechanical translation leads to faster data acquisition speed in FD-OCT. The instantaneous current generated in an FD-OCT detection system by incoming light is a function dependent on the source wavelength sampled at a particular instance. The acquired data is transformed into axial scan information (A-scan) by an inverse Fourier transform [6]. Fourier Dormain-OCT consists of two primary methods, spectral dormain and swept source OCT. The two variants are abbreviated as SD and SS domain OCT, respectively.

The Spectral domain OCT employs principle of Michelson-type interferometry that utilizes a static reference mirror. The generated interference signal is detected and the dual returning beams are recombined to form an interference pattern at the beam splitter. At this point a diffraction grating disperses the beam which is detected by a high-speed charge-couple device (CCD) camera. The generated interference pattern detected by the line camera produces an array that results in obtaining tissue reflectivity as a depth function. The detection rate of the line sensor defines the acquisition speed of such systems [7]. Interference patterns are dispersed quite rapidly before detection in spectral domain OCT while in the Swept source OCT a laser with a limited spectral line within the available bandwidth of the source scan the tissues in a regulated way. Subsequently, the mirror reflected reference beam generates an interference pattern with the light backscattered by the tissue and this is identified by the detector. Point detection is one advantage that swept source has over spectral domain OCT because of its higher signal-to-noise ratio when compared to line detectors [8]. Fourier domain OCT has reduced artifacts and faster scan acquisition time which permits three dimensional image construction [9]. High reflectivity tissues are depicted in red, medium yellow to green while low appears as blue to black.

The limitations of OCT include poor signal strength in the presence of opacity in the ocular media which prevents data acquisition. Patients with macular problems that reduced the central vision may have difficulty fixating on the target. Motion artifacts can give rise to false observations, and such artifacts are commoner in eyes with underlying pathology [10]. The technology is expensive and not available in most tertiary hospitals in the sub-Saharan African region. The few available ones are mainly located in urban centers away from vast majority in rural communities. OCT scan is not covered by the health insurance scheme which in any way is only available to the few working in regular public/private sectors.

2. OCT in glaucoma

Glaucoma is the second leading cause of blindness [11]. The standard method of diagnosis is based on clinical evaluation of characteristic optic nerve damage and the visual field changes detected by standard automated perimetry (SAP). OCT provides additional evaluation and assessment for monitoring glaucoma progression thought it may not be of much value in patients with advanced disease. Visual field changes are not detected in early stages of glaucoma due to the functional overlapping pattern and integration of the visual system which compensate for and to some extent mask early damage. A 6 mm^3 scan centered on the disk provides graphic and quantifiable retinal thickness measurements in addition to providing an objective calculation of the cupping by giving details of the extent of vertical cup-to-disk ratio. Effective management requires detection of early changes in glaucoma even before development of detectable

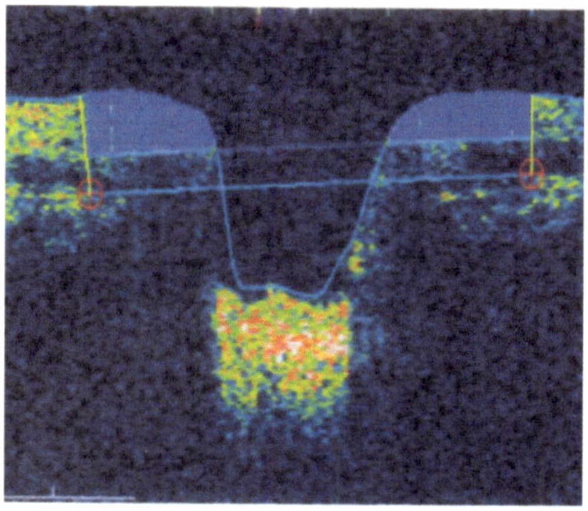

Figure 1.
OCT illustration of glaucomatous optic disk cupping.

visual field defects as neural damage may precede visual field defects by many years. Significant differences in RNFL thickness have been observed to occur up to 8 years before detectable visual field defects [12]. Thus OCT is quite useful in identifying changes in retinal nerve fiber layer (RNFL) thickness, the optic nerve head structure (ONH), and the macular ganglion cell complex (GCC). A 3.46 mm para-papillary scan entered on the optic nerve head evaluates RNFL thickness in all the quadrants and is useful in assessment and monitoring of glaucoma progression. In most instances, the RNFL thickness is highest in the inferior quadrant followed by superior, nasal, and temporal quadrants in that order (ISNT rule) [13]. Analysis of the RNFL and inner macular thickness has provided additional means of determining glaucomatous optic nerve damage and progression [14]. There is paucity of normative RNFL data in sub-Saharan Africa though some reports indicate an RNFL average of 110 and 104.17 μm, respectively [15, 16]. RNFL below 100 μm is suspect, less than 90 μm requires full glaucoma workup, and values less than 70 μm are not unusual at the time of glaucoma diagnosis. Reduction of the average thickness within certain time frame can be an indicator of progression in addition to perimetric changes. **Figure 1** shows glaucoma optic nerve damage on OCT.

3. OCT in macular diseases

The macula serves as the most acute visual function, and conventional assessment includes ophthalmoscopy and slit lamp evaluation in conjunction with contact and noncontact retinal lenses. Naked eye assessment can however not be compared with quantifiable OCT analysis. Fast macular scan protocol can be employed to provide graphic image of the state of the macula. Macular scan results can be displayed as numeric data or as false color display form. Normative data in Africans is not largely available though a study indicates macular thickness and volume of 149.58 and 6.79 μm^3, respectively [17]. Central macular thickness above 200 μm is uncommon in healthy eyes and deserves further evaluation even when the vision is not significantly affected. Macular thickness measurements in diabetic macular edema are based on criteria definition of existing standard protocol. Macular thickness measurement below 110 μm is rarely observed in normal eyes. Disorders of the macula include diabetic maculopathy and other forms of acquired maculopathy such as age-related macular degeneration. A survey report indicated diabetic retinopathy (DR) to be a cause of blindness and visual impairment despite some patients being

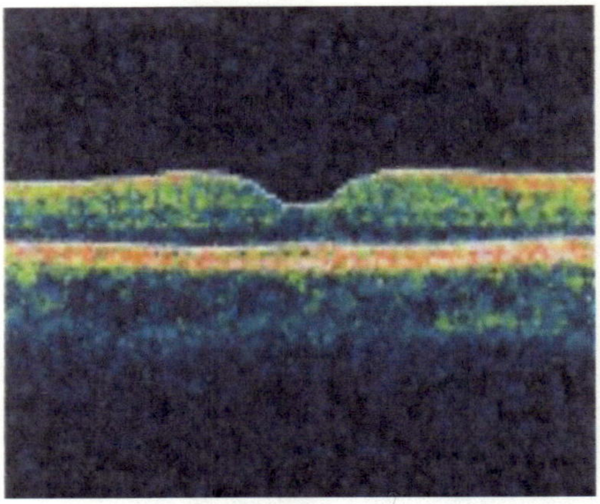

Figure 2.
OCT showing normal macular scan.

unaware of their diabetic status [18, 19]. DR rivals cataract and glaucoma as a cause of visual impairment in an institution-based study of diabetic patients [20]. Diabetic cystoid macular edema (CME), diffuse thickening, and serous detachment can objectively be measured with OCT [21, 22]. OCT demonstrates retinal thickening and cystoid spaces in the presence of CME. As OCT was not in use during the ETDRS, [23] clinically significant macular edema was defined by the presence of retinal thickening within 500 μm of fovea or hard exudates within 500 μm of the fovea or retinal thickening more than one disk diameter any part of which is within a disk diameter of the fovea [24]. OCT has been demonstrated to quantify the extent of CSME at diagnosis even more accurately than clinical fundal assessment and can serve in determining response to treatment applied. **Figure 2** shows a normal OCT macular scan, and **Figure 3** shows cystoid spaces in macular edema. Likewise OCT can be used to monitor resolution of CME with appropriate treatment.

Age-related macular degeneration (ARMD) is a group of primary disorders of the retina which are emerging as a significant cause of visual impairment in developed countries. With change in lifestyle, the disease is becoming common even in developing countries though a population survey report showed it was not a significant cause of visual impairment [17]. ARMD has been classified into dry (non-exudative) and wet (exudative) types. The dry type is the most common, and geographic atrophy is the manifestation of the late stage of the disease. The International Age Related

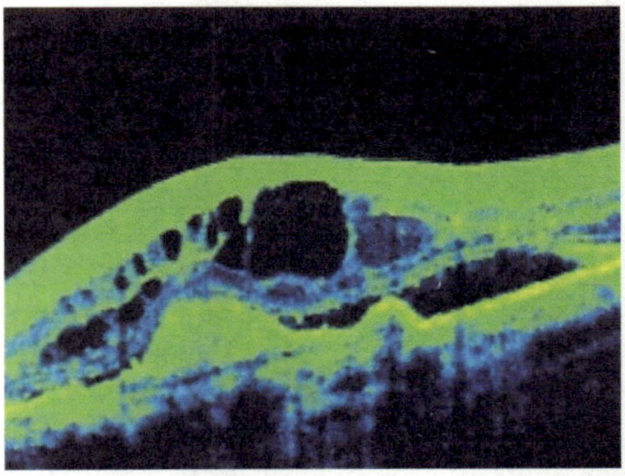

Figure 3.
Clinically significant macular edema.

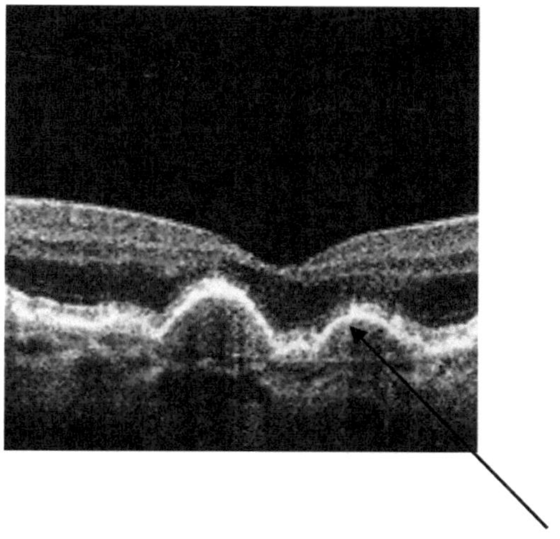

Figure 4.
OCT features of macula drusen.

Maculopathy Epidemiological Study Group (IARMESG) has classified the disease further age-related maculopathy (ARM) into early (medium to large drusen, retinal pigment epithelium (RP) hyperpigmentation and/or hypopigmentation). **Figure 4** shows drusen on OCT scan. Advanced AMD is characterized by geographic atrophy (**Figure 5**) and/or choroidal neovascularization. SD-OCT has been demonstrated to quantify the volume of drusen and thus monitor progression [25]. OCT has been demonstrated to be useful in estimating photoreceptor loss, quantifying the extent, and providing insight as to the structural damage leading to enlargement and progression of geographic atrophy in non-neovascular AMD [26, 27]. Retinal pigment epithelium (RPE) detachment arises from dysfunction of the normal physiologic factors that ensures its adhesion to Bruch's membrane. The separation occurs between the basement membrane of the RPE and the inner collagenous layer of Bruch's membrane which become thickened and dysfunctional. The separation appears as an optically empty space on OCT (**Figure 6**). OCT can distinguish two

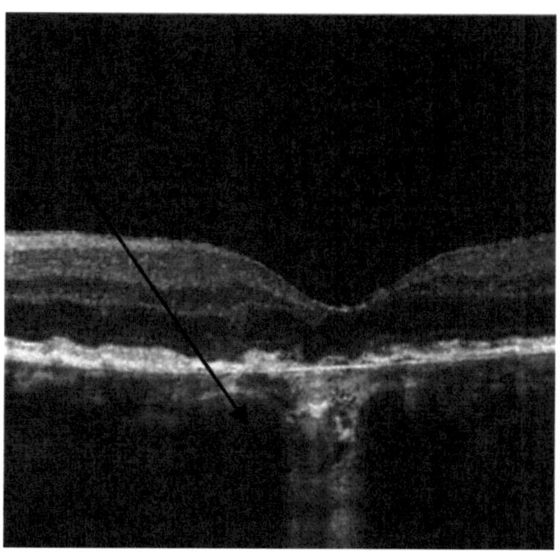

Figure 5.
OCT features of geographic atrophy (source: www.octscans.com).

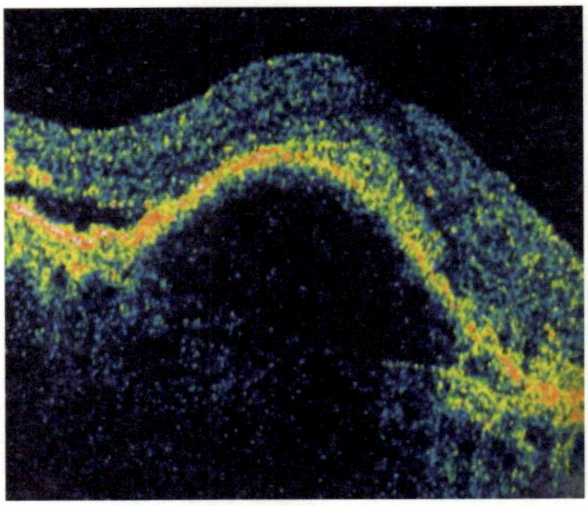

Figure 6.
Retinal pigment epithelial detaachment showing Optically empty space between Bruch's membrane and separated RPE.

broad types of RPE detachment, thus aiding in making accurate diagnosis [28]. Wet AMD is associated with choroidal neovascularization (CNV). The blood vessels arise from the choriocapillaris and break through Bruch's membrane. CNV membrane (**Figure 7**) can remain in the sub RPE or even extend into the subretinal space. Fundal fluorescein angiography (FFA) is the primary investigation in diagnosis of suspected CNV. The role of OCT is in providing quantifiable monitoring of response to treatment. OCT shows increased thickness and fragmentation of the high reflectivity RPE and choriocapillaris. Improvement in data acquisition and 3-D imaging in SD-OCT provides more detailed images leading to higher and earlier detection of CNV when compared to time-domain technology [29]. Combined OCT angiography provides additional value in diagnosis and monitoring of the impact of treatment in wet ARM.

Macular hole is one of the age-related causes of vision loss, and studies have shown that macular hole is not uncommon in sub-Saharan Africans [30, 31]. Population incidence of 6.8–8.69 has been reported in the Unites States [32]. Occult, lamellar, full-thickness holes, and complete posterior vitreous detachment (PVD) can accurately be quantified on OCT. Full-thickness hole is identified including a pseudo operculum where present. OCT is used for characterization of macular

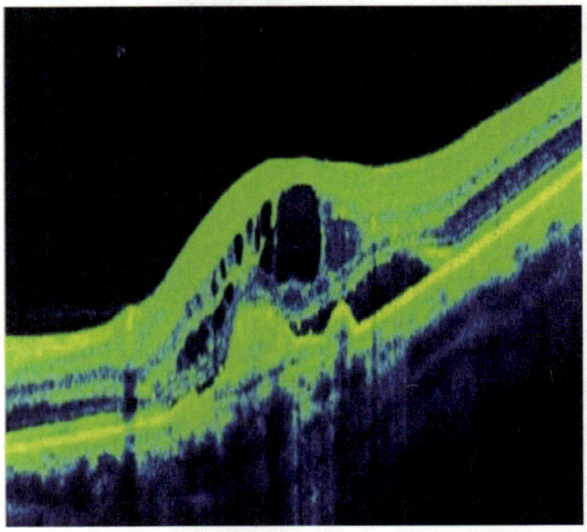

Figure 7.
OCT showing choroidal neovascularization.

holes and to visualize persistent retinal abnormalities which were observed despite achieving anatomical closure [32, 33].

4. Impact of OCT on glaucoma and diabetic macular edema

OCT has aided the ophthalmologist in early detection and provides a more objective monitoring tool in glaucoma management in sub-Saharan Africa. This is achieved by effective detection of RNFL loss and evaluation of the differential measurements in the four quadrants to detect deviation from normal (normal RNFL thickness declines measurement in this order: inferior, superior, medial, and temporal quadrants—ISN'T rule). OCT RNFL can be utilized alone or better in combination with standard automated perimetry in monitoring for stabilization or deterioration of glaucomatous optic neuropathy over time. This will enable the clinician to counsel the patient using objective criteria and modify the treatment to achieve goal of effective glaucoma control. OCT gives accurate central macular thickness measurement and thus provides effective and early detection of clinically significant diabetic macular edema. The impact of laser and/or intravitreal anti-VEGF on treatment of proliferative diabetic retinopathy and macular edema can be determined.

5. Conclusion

OCT is still a relatively new technology in the diagnosis and monitoring of glaucoma and macular diseases in the region. Older models are available in few centers and clinicians have limited access. By the poor income of most sub-Saharan Africans, OCT scan is expensive. Most of the machines have no provision for digital data retrieval, thus making research work on impact of the technology more difficult. Normative data on various parameters have to be locally generated in order to make more objective decision when there is variation from normal. In few countries with limited health insurance services (which only cover workers in the national public service), OCT is exempted as has to be paid for as out-of-pocket expense, thus further limited access to the vast population. A public-private partnership could enhance availability to the underserved population.

Acknowledgement

The author would like to appreciate the management of Bayero University, Kano, Nigeria, for providing an enabling academic environment.

Conflict of interest

None.

Author details

Lawan Abdu
Department of Ophthalmology, Faculty of Clinical Sciences, College of Health Sciences, Bayero University Kano, Nigeria

*Address all correspondence to: lawal1966@yahoo.com

References

[1] Dan PP, Lin-P'ing CS, Costel F, Youxin M, Shoude C, John D, et al. Optical coherence tomography: Fundamental principles, instrumental designs and biomedical applications. Biophysical Reviews. 2011;**3**(3):155

[2] Huang D, Swanson EA, Lin CP, Schuman JS, Stinson WG, Chang W, et al. Optical coherence tomography. Science. 1991;**254**:1178-1181

[3] Muna B, Sharan S, Mohana KP, Ramya S. Optical coherence tomography: A guide to interpretation of common macular diseases. Indian Journal of Ophthalmology. 2018;**66**(1):20-35

[4] J Fernando A, Andres FL, Juan DA, Martin AS, Fernando AA. Clinical applications of optical coherence tomography in the posterior pole: The 2011 José Manuel Espino Lecture—Part II. Clinical Ophthalmology. 2013;**7**:2181-2206

[5] Fercher AF, Hitzenberger CK, Kamp G, Elzaint SY. Measurement of intra ocular distance by back scattering spectral interferometry. Optics Communication. 1995;**117**:43-48

[6] Hauster G, Lindner MW. "Coherence radar" and "spectral radar"—New tools for dermatological diagnosis. Journal of Biomedical Optics. 1998;**3**(1):21-31

[7] Wojtkowski M, Leitgeb R, Kowalczyk A, Bajroszewki T, Fercher AF. In vivo retinal imaging by Fourier dormain optical coherence tomography. Journal of Biomedical Optics. 2002;**7**(93):457-463

[8] Golubovic B, Bouma BE, Teomey GJ, Fujimoto JG. Optical frequency-dormain reflectometry using rapid wavelenghth tuning Cr4: Forsterite laser. Optics Letters. 1997;**22**(22):1704-1706

[9] Dainty C, Podoleanu A. Evaluation of the signal noise ratio enhancement of SS-OCT versus TD-OCT using full field interferometer. Proceedings of SPIE. 2009;**7168**:71682K. DOI: 10.1117/12.809043

[10] Ghasemi FK, Al-Sheikh M, Akil H, Sadda SR. Image artefacts in swept-source optical coherence tomography angiography. The British Journal of Ophthalmology. Ophthalmol. 2017;**101**(5):564-568

[11] Quigley HA, Broman AT. The number of people with glaucoma worldwide 2010 and 2020. The British Journal of Ophthalmology. 2006;**90**(3):262-267

[12] Kuang TM, Zhang C, Zangwill LM, Weinreb RN, Medeiros FA. Estimating lead time gained by optical coherence tomography in detecting glaucoma before development of visual field defects. Ophthalmology. 2015;**122**(10):2002-2009

[13] Alasil T, Wang K, Keane PA, Lee H, Baniasadi N, de Boer JF, et al. Analysis of normal retinal nerve fiber layer thickness by age, sex, and race using spectral domain optical coherence tomography. Journal of Glaucoma. 2013;**22**(7):532-541

[14] Leung CK. Diagnosing glaucoma progression with optical coherence tomography. Current Opinion in Ophthalmology. 2014;**25**(2):104-111

[15] Khathutshelo PM, Olalekan AO. Retinal nerve fiber layer thickness values and their associations with ocular and systemic parameters in Black South Africans. African Health Sciences. 2016;**16**(4):1188-1194

[16] Rabi YS, Lawan A, Victoria P. Retinal nerve fiber layer thickness measurements of normal Northern

Nigerian adults using optical coherence tomography. Annals of African Medicine. 2016;**15**(2):52-57

[17] Lawan A, Rabi YS. Macular volume and central foveal thickness measurements in normal eyes of healthy Nigerian Adults using optical coherence tomography. Annals of African Medicine. 2014;**13**(3):134-137

[18] Mohammed MA, Selvaraj S, Gudlavalleti VS, Murthy G, Clare G, Tafida A, et al. Causes of blindness and visual impairment in Nigeria: The Nigeria national blindness and visual impairment survey. Investigative Ophthalmology & Visual Science. 2009;**50**:4114-4120

[19] Fatima K, Abubakar T, Selvaraj S, Gudlavalleti VS, Murthy G, Tunde P, et al. Prevalence and risk factors for diabetes and diabetic retinopathy: Results from the Nigeria national blindness and visual impairment survey. BMC Public Health. 2014;**14**:1299

[20] Abdu L, Tijjani BM. Pattern of diabetic retinopathy in Kano, Nigeria. Annals of African Medicine. 2012;**11**(2):75-79

[21] Charlotte S, Birgit S, Nicolai L, Michael L, Henrik LA. Diabetic macular edema assessed with optical coherence tomography and stereo fundus photography. Investigative Ophthalmology & Visual Science. 2002;**43**(1):241-245

[22] Kim BY, Smith SD, Kaiser PK. Optical coherence tomography patterns of diabetic macular edema. American Journal of Ophthalmology. 2006;**142**(3):405-412

[23] Early Treatment Diabetic Retinopathy Study Research (ETDRS) Group. Treatment techniques and clinical guidelines for photocoagulation of diabetic macular edema. Early treatment diabetic retinopathy study report number 2. Ophthalmology. 1987;**94**:761-774

[24] Early Treatment Diabetic Retinopathy Study Research Group. Photocoagulation for diabetic macular edema. Early treatment diabetic retinopathy study report number 1. Archives of Ophthalmology. 1985;**103**:1796-1806

[25] Giovanni G, Fenghua W, Philip JR, Zohar Y, Ninel ZG, Brandon JL, et al. Spectral domain optical coherence tomography imaging of drusen in nonexudative age-related macular degeneration. Ophthalmology. 2011;**118**(7):1373-1379

[26] Srilaxmi B, Felix YC, Anjum K, Sandra SS, Joseph AI, Cynthia AT. Spectral domain optical coherence tomography imaging of geographic atrophy margins. Ophthalmology. 2009;**116**(9):1762-1769

[27] Zohar Y, Philip JR, Giovanni G, William JF, Manuel F, Brandon JL, et al. Progression of geographic atrophy in age-related macular degeneration imaged with spectral domain optical coherence tomography. Ophthalmology. 2011;**118**(4):679-686

[28] Yoshida M, Abe T, Kano T, Tumai M. Two types of optical coherence tomography images of retinal pigment epithelial detachment with different prognosis. British Journal of Ophthalmology. 2002;**86**:737-739

[29] Caio VR, Lauren B, Jay SD. The role of spectral-domain OCT in the diagnosis and management of neovascular age-related macular degeneration. Ophthalmic Surgery, Lasers & Imaging. 2011;**42**:S56-S66

[30] Uhumwangho OM, Itina EI. Retinal diseases in a tertiary hospital in southern Nigeria. Journal of the West African College of Surgeons. 2015;**5**(2):1-16

[31] Oluleye TS, Ajaiyeogba AI. Retinal diseases in Ibadan. Eye. 2006;**20**:1461-1463

[32] Hee MR, Puliafito CA, Wong C, Duker JS, Reichel E, Schuman JS, et al. Optical coherence tomography of macular holes. Ophthalmology. 1995;**102**(5):748-756

[33] Tony HK, Andre JW, James GF, Annie C, Adam HR, Caroline RB, et al. Ultrahigh-resolution optical coherence tomography of surgically closed macular holes. Archives of Ophthalmology. 2006;**124**(6):827-836

Chapter 3

Topical NSAIDs in Prevention of Postcataract Macular Edema

Ahmed Alnagdy, Ahmed M. Eissa and Amr El-Kannishy

Abstract

Postoperative macular edema is considered one cause of diminished vision after cataract surgery. It was approved that inflammatory mediators especially prostaglandins play a key role in macular edema formation especially in the presence of risk factors that affect blood-retinal barrier such as diabetes, uveitis, tear of posterior capsule, and vitreous loss. So, anti-inflammatory medications like corticosteroids and NSAIDs are the cornerstone of macular edema managements. In spite of using corticosteroids as gold standard for treatment of ocular inflammation, they cannot be used for prolonged period due to associated adverse effects. Lastly, there were many studies about benefits of NSAIDs in management and prevention of macular edema to avoid the side effects of corticosteroids.

Keywords: NSAIDs, macular edema, phacoemulsification, cataract, blood-retinal barrier

1. Introduction

Macula is an important part of the retina, which is responsible for color vision, contrast sensitivity, sharp vision, communications and interpersonal relationships [1].

Macular thickening is well-known postoperative complication after cataract surgery, even with uncomplicated small incision phacoemulsification surgery. Subclinical cystoid macular edema (CME) is diagnosed with fluorescein angiography as leakage from perifoveal dilated capillaries without visual acuity affection [2]. Although fluorescein angiography is considered gold standard for diagnosis of macular edema, quantification of fluorescein leakage is difficult. Optical coherence tomography (OCT) nowadays has an upper hand in diagnosis of macular edema because of its advantages as a noninvasive device and can detect macular edema quantitatively and qualitatively [3].

Clinical CME can be identified on biomicroscopic examination and is associated with decreased visual acuity [4].

The pathogenesis of CME is disruption of blood-retinal barrier (BRB) by inflammatory mediators generated through several cascades as a result of surgical trauma to iris, ciliary body, or lens epithelial cells. Also, preexisting ocular conditions such as diabetes, hypertension, and uveitis, which affect BRB, can increase risk of CME [5].

The blood-retinal barrier in diabetic eyes is impaired to a variable degree, which plays a role in development of postoperative CME. CME in diabetic patients is affected by many factors including duration, severity of the disease, presence of retinopathy, and previous treatment with photocoagulation [6]. Total ophthalmic payments were documented to be 47% higher in patients who developed postoperative CME [7]. So, prophylactic prevention or even decreased CME severity is cost savings, particularly among diabetic patients.

2. Macular anatomy and physiology

Being the main part of clear vision, the macula is located in the heart of the retina between upper and lower arcades measured about 4.5–6 mm in diameter. It can be divided into central fovea, surrounded by parafovea and outer perifovea (**Figure 1**) [8].

- Retinal vascular plexus was described simply into two planes: inner one at ganglion cell layer and outer plexus at inner nuclear layer [9] (**Figure 2**).

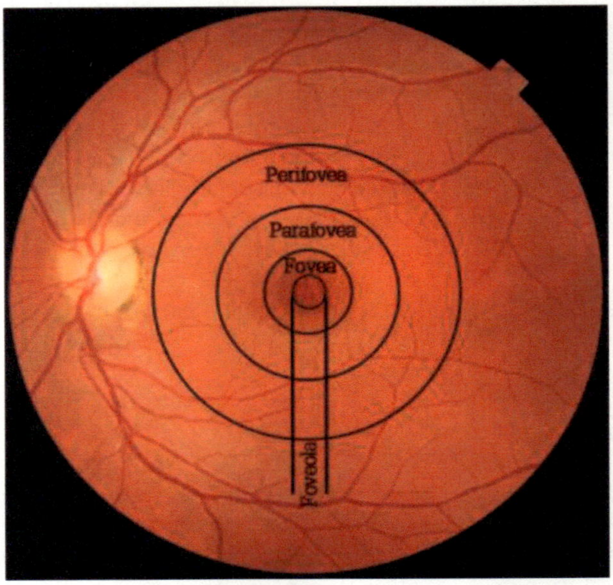

Figure 1.
Parts of the macula from inside to outside: foveola, fovea, parafovea, and perifovea [8].

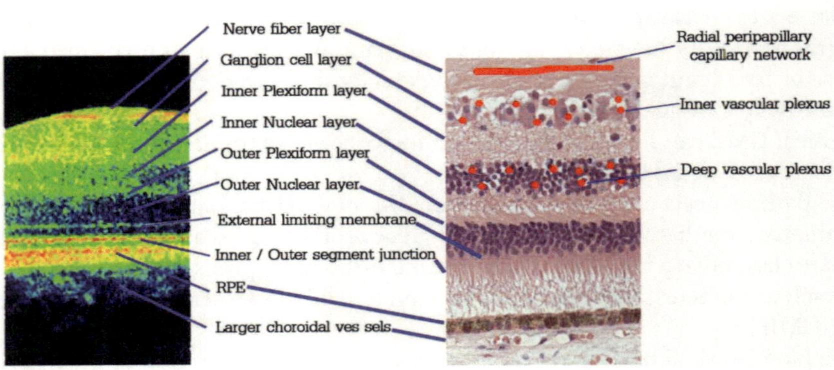

Figure 2.
Vascular plexus position in layers of retina: inner vascular plexus in ganglion cell layer and deep vascular plexus in inner nuclear layer [9].

- As a whole, the retina blood supply is divided into outer part supplied by choriocapillaris and inner part supplied by retinal vascular plexus branch of posterior ciliary arteries [10].

3. The blood-retinal barrier

The blood-retinal barrier (BRB) is a barrier that physiologically establishes and maintains specific substrate and ion concentrations to allow proper neural function. BRB regulates flux of substances in retina such as ion, protein, and water and also regulates infiltration of immune competent cells and blood toxins. BRB is formed at two levels, inner and outer BRB. The inner one is composed of tight junctions between retinal vascular endothelial cells. The outer barrier is composed of tight junction between retinal pigment epithelium cells [11].

Pericytes secrete angiopoietin 1, which induces tight junction protein expression to support endothelial cells barrier [12].

3.1 Tight junction

Tight junction is mainly apical junctional complex, which has a barrier function against solute flux and movement of proteins and lipids into retinal parenchyma. This junction is showed as transmembrane proteins and junctional adhesion molecule (JAM) [13].

3.2 Adherens junction

Adherens junction is second barrier beneath the tight junction. This junction is important for development of the barrier as it affects formation of tight junction [14].

Tight junction: Transmembrane proteins claudins, occludin, and junctional adhesion molecule (JAM) connected with scaffolding protein ZO to actin.

Adherens junction: Vascular endothelial (VE) cadherin connected to actin through complex of β-catenin, α-catenin, and vinculin.

4. Pathophysiology

The macula is responsible for central 30 degrees of sharp vision with color vision, interpersonal relationships, communications, and contrast sensitivity [1]. The retina is very sensitive to fluctuation in blood oxygen levels and intraocular changes, as it consumes oxygen more than other tissues, being highly active tissue. Microchanges not felt by patient visual acuity are also not seen by inspection ophthalmoscopy examination [15].

It has been reported that clinical affection due to CME after uneventful phacoemulsification is between 0 and 9%. Furthermore, clinical affection between 9.1 and 20.4% with angiographic leakage is reported [16]. Interruption of blood-retinal barrier is the most accepted explanation of postoperative macular edema, which causes macular thickening. Surgical trauma disrupts the blood-aqueous barrier, release of prostaglandins, and increase of perifoveal capillaries' permeability of liquid in extracellular spaces, which cause macular thickening and CME [17]. The pathophysiology of these macular changes may be considered consecutively as follows: (1) release of inflammatory mediators into anterior chamber produced by surgical procedures; (2) removal of normally lens barrier, which separate posterior segment from anterior segment; (3) local effect of inflammatory mediators on macular area; and (4) anterior displacement of vitreous leading to increase traction on macula [18].

Recently, being noninvasive, OCT has been established to be the main method for examining retinal architecture [19]. OCT can measure microhistological retinal changes in difference to fluorescein angiography, which detects it as a leakage that cannot be detected by biomicroscopy [20]. It was reported that subclinical increase in retinal thickness and volume can be found in the early course postoperatively at 4 weeks after phacoemulsification [21].

5. Nonsteroidal anti-inflammatory drugs

Surgical trauma stimulates arachidonic acid cascade, which stimulates phospholipase A2 enzyme to release arachidonic acid from membrane phospholipids and produces inflammatory mediators including prostaglandins (PGs) and leukotriene by activation of cyclooxygenase (COX) enzymes. COX-1 and COX-2 isoforms are believed to be the primary mediator of ocular inflammation. PG is an important mediator of postoperative complications, associated with symptoms including pain, ciliary injection, cystoid macular edema, impaired vision, and intraoperative miosis [22].

So, treatment of ocular inflammation depends mainly on stopping of arachidonic cascades by corticosteroids and nonsteroidal anti-inflammatory drugs (NSAIDs). Corticosteroids inhibit the activity of phospholipase A2 enzyme, but NSAIDs inhibit PGs synthesis irreversibly and nonspecifically by direct inhibition of COX-1 and COX-2 activity [23] (**Figure 3**).

5.1 Corticosteroids

In spite of using corticosteroids as gold standard for treatment of ocular inflammation, they cannot be used for prolonged period due to associated adverse effects.

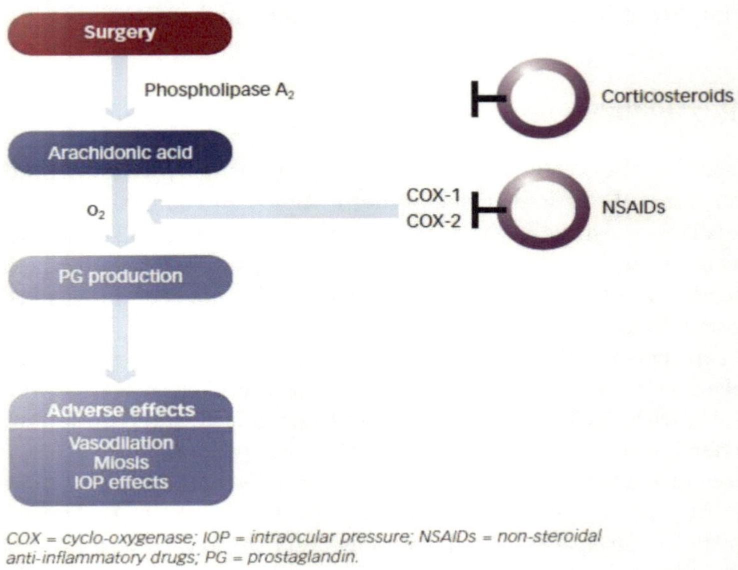

Figure 3.
Action of corticosteroid and NSAIDs on arachidonic acid cascade [23].

Side effects of corticosteroids include increased susceptibility to infections as a result of suppression of host immune response, retardation of corneal wound healing, and increased intraocular pressure (IOP) [24].

5.2 Nonsteroidal anti-inflammatory drugs

NSAIDs are considered as safety option used for treatment of ocular inflammation. NSAIDs inhibit COX activity patently by several chemically heterogeneous classes [25].

Currently, the uses of topical NSAIDs in ophthalmology to reduce pain and discomfort after cataract and refractive surgery prevent intraoperative miosis during cataract surgery and manage postoperative inflammation (**Table 1**) and are also reported to have a role in prevention of CME after cataract surgery [25, 27].

NSAIDs have beneficial effects over corticosteroids including analgesia effect, maintaining pupillary dilatation if used preoperatively (**Figure 4**), and also reduce the risk of secondary infections and increased IOP [25].

5.3 Pharmacokinetics

Diclofenac: Plasma levels reached (10 ng/mL) during a 4 hours period after instillation of two drops in each eye [29].

Flurbiprofen: No information about systemic absorption was approved.

Ketorolac: The use of ketorolac in 26 patients with one drop in each eye three times daily resulted in 5/26 (= 19.2%) with detectable plasma level of ketorolac (10.7–22.5 ng/mL) after 10 days.

Bromfenac: After topical administration, plasma level is expected to be below the detectable limit (50 ng/mL).

Nepafenac: It is an inactive prodrug, which penetrates corneal epithelium and is converted by ocular tissue hydrolases to active form amfenac. Plasma levels of bromfenac and amfenac were detected 2–3 hours in most patients after installation of nepafenac in both eyes but with low plasma level.

Drug	Indications	
Diclofenac sodium	Management of postoperative inflammation in patients after cataract extraction Decrease of pain and photophobia in patients after corneal refractive surgery	
Flurbiprofen sodium	Maintenance of intraoperative pupil dilatation	
Ketorolac tromethamine	(0.5%)	Temporary relief of ocular itching associated with seasonal allergic conjunctivitis Management of postoperative inflammation in patients after cataract extraction
	(0.4%)	Decrease of ocular pain and burning/stinging in patients undergoing corneal refractive surgery
	(0.45%) (0.5%)	Reduction of ocular pain and inflammation associated with/following cataract surgery
Bromfenac sodium	Management of postoperative inflammation and pain after cataract surgery	
Nepafenac	Management of inflammation and pain associated with cataract surgery	

Table 1.
Ophthalmic NSAIDs' FDA-approved indications [26].

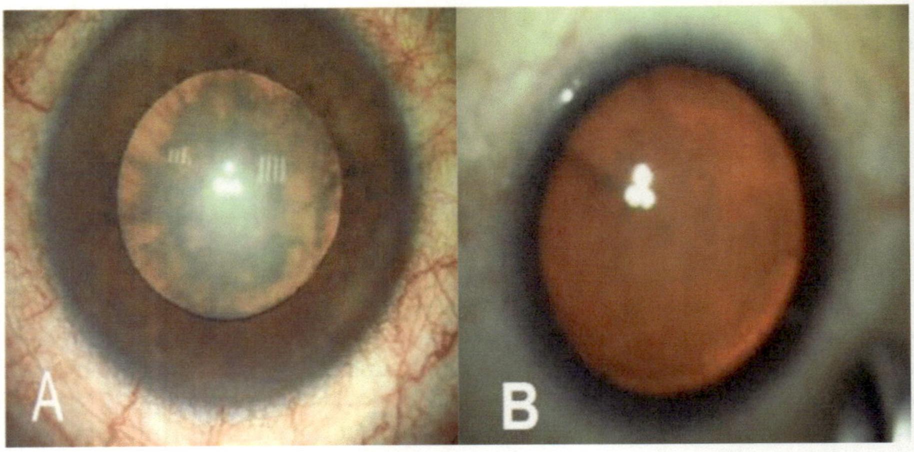

Figure 4.
Comparing pupil poor dilatation in control group (A) and full dilated pupil with NSAIDs (B) [28].

5.4. Limitation of NSAIDs

Topical NSAIDs contain some warnings, which include the following:

1. Prolonged bleeding time [30].

2. Cross-sensitivity with phenyl acetic acid derivatives, acetylsalicylic acid, and other NSAIDs [31].

3. Delay wound healing mainly if used in combination with corticosteroids [32].

4. Topical NSAIDs may cause ocular surface toxicity especially in patients having dry eye syndrome, corneal denervation, corneal epithelial defects, or diabetes [33].

6. Discussion

In the last few years, there were many studies using NSAIDs to prevent postoperative CME in different situations. In **Table 2**, some studies focus on the effect of NSAIDs in prevention of postoperative CME in diabetic patients. All of them approved significant low macular thickening in diabetic patients receiving NSAID bromfenac only [34], classical postoperative steroid regimen in addition of nepafenac [35] or either nepafenac or ketorolac with classical postoperative steroid regimen [28].

Other studies documented the effect of NSAIDs in a mixed population (nondiabetic and diabetic patients) without cystoid macular edema preoperatively and with no predisposing factors for developing cystoid macular edema (**Table 3**). Some studies documented that topical steroid medication may not be absolutely essential after uneventful cataract surgery [37, 44]. Topical nonsteroidal started 1 day before surgery and continued for 1 month by Almeida et al. [37], while Nishino et al. [44] started medication postoperatively and continued for 1 month. On the other hand, many studies approved the significant importance of topical NSAIDs in prevention of macular edema [36, 38–43, 45, 46]. topical ketorolac had more effect in decreasing macular edema than prednisolone only, if started 2 days before surgery and continued for 1 month postoperatively in combination with

Study	Number	Groups	Follow-up	Conclusion
Endo et al. [34]	62 (26 patients with nonproliferative diabetic retinopathy)	1. Bromfenac (n = 31) (16 with NPDR) 2. Steroidal solution (n = 31) (11 with NPDR)	OCT 6 weeks	The perifoveal values were significantly lower in the bromfenac group
Singh et al. [35]	263 patients with nonproliferative diabetic retinopathy	1. Nepafenac (n = 125) 2. Vehicle (n = 126)	OCT 90 days	Significantly lower percentage of patients in the nepafenac group developed macular edema
Alnagdy et al. [28]	80 without diabetic retinopathy	1. Placebo group + prednisolone 2. Nepafenac 0.1% + prednisolone 3. Ketorolac 0.4% + prednisolone	OCT 3 months	Perioperative NSAIDs reduce the frequency and severity of CME in diabetic eyes following cataract surgery

Table 2.
Clinical trials using ophthalmic NSAIDs to prevent postoperative macular edema in diabetic patients without cystoid macular edema preoperatively and with no predisposing factors for developing cystoid macular edema.

Study	Number	Groups	Follow-up	Conclusion
Almeida et al. [36]	106	1. Prednisolone 1% 2. Prednisolone 1% + ketorolac 0.5%	OCT 1 month	After cataract surgery, ketorolac 0.5% effectively decreases postoperative macular edema
Almeida et al. [37]	193	1. Prednisolone 1% 2. Prednisolone 1% + nepafenac 0.1% 3. Prednisolone 1% + ketorolac 0.5% (1 day before surgery for 1 month postoperative)	OCT 1 month	There was no difference in macular volume between the placebo, ketorolac, and nepafenac
Cable et al. [38]	20 diabetic patients without edema could be enrolled	1. Prednisolone + bromfenac 2. Prednisolone + nepafenac	OCT 6 weeks	Postoperative bromfenac showed a trend toward improved vision, less retinal thickening, and more stable macular volumes overall
Cervantes-Coste et al. [39]	60 excluding proliferative DR, macular edema, uncontrolled DM	1. Dexamethasone 2. Dexamethasone + nepafenac	OCT 6 weeks	Nepafenac has a rule in reducing macular edema after cataract surgery and in maintaining intraoperative mydriasis
Rossetti et al. 1996 [40]	88	1. Diclofenac 2. Placebo	Ocular inflammation and FFA and visual acuity 6 months	Diclofenac eye drops effectively reduced incidence of angiographic CME and ocular inflammation after cataract surgery

Study	Number	Groups	Follow-up	Conclusion
Miyake et al. [41]	118 without complications from diabetes mellitus	1. Fluorometholone 2. Diclofenac	Fundus fluorescein angiography (FFA) 8 weeks	Diclofenac was effective in prevention of CME following cataract surgery
Miyake et al. [42]	62	1. Fluorometholone 2. Diclofenac	FFA 5 weeks	Diclofenac was more effective than fluorometholone in preventing cystoid macular edema
Miyake et al. [43]	60	1. Fluorometholone 2. Nepafenac	OCT 5 weeks	Nepafenac was more effective than fluorometholone in preventing cystoid macular edema
Nishino et al. [44]	21	1. Bromfenac 2. Fluorometholone	FFA 1 month	Topical steroid medication may not be absolutely essential after uneventful phacoemulsification
Weber et al. [45]	123	1. Indomethacin 0.1% 2. Ketorolac 0.5%	OCT 90 days	Indomethacin 0.1% had the same effect as ketorolac 0.5% at first day postoperative and more effective than ketorolac 0.5% at first week in treating ocular inflammation after uncomplicated cataract surgery. There was no change from baseline in retinal thickness in two groups
Wittpenn et al. [46]	546	1. Ketorolac 0.4% (only 1 hour prior to surgery) + prednisolone for 1 month 2. Ketorolac 0.4 + prednisolone for 1 month	OCT 4–6 weeks	Perioperative ketorolac to postoperative prednisolone significantly reduces the macular thickening after cataract surgery

Table 3.
Clinical trials using ophthalmic NSAIDs to prevent postoperative macular edema in a mixed population (nondiabetic and diabetic patients) without cystoid macular edema preoperatively and with no predisposing factors for developing cystoid macular edema.

prednisolone had more effect in decreasing macular edema in comparison to postoperative topical prednisolone alone [36]. Wittpenn et al. approved that starting ketorolac 1 hour before surgery had significant effects in preventing macular edema [46]. Cervantes-Coste et al. documented that diclofenac effectively maintains mydriasis and decreases macular thickness [39]. Also, diclofenac eye drops in Rossetti et al. effectively reduced incidence of angiographic CME and ocular inflammation after cataract surgery [40], while Miyake et al. suggested that diclofenac effectively decreases CME in comparison to fluorometholone [41] and also approved its effect in preventing chronological change in choroidal blood flow and disruption of the blood-aqueous barrier [42]. In 2011, there was another study by

Miyake et al. which approved that nepafenac was more effective than fluorometholone in preventing cystoid macular edema [43]. In other hand, some studies compared the effect of different NSAIDs similar to the study by Cable et al. who suggested that bromfenac is more effective than nepafenac [38] and Weber et al. who suggested that there was no change from baseline in retinal thickness between indomethacin group and ketorolac group.

Nondiabetic patients who have undergone cataract surgery without preoperative macular edema and with no predisposing factors for developing cystoid macular edema were enrolled in studies in **Table 4**. In glaucoma patients after cataract surgery, Miyake et al. approved that diclofenac seems to prevent macular edema formation enhanced by latanoprost therapy [49], and timolol and its preservative benzalkonium chloride [50].

Study	Number	Groups	Follow-up	Conclusion
Donnenfeld et al. [47]	100	1. Prednisolone acetate 2. Ketorolac (3 days preoperative and 3 weeks postoperative) + prednisolone 3. Ketorolac (1 day preoperative and 3 weeks postoperative) + prednisolone 4. Ketorolac (1 hour preoperative and 3 weeks postoperative) + prednisolone	OCT 3 months	The preoperative use of ketorolac tromethamine 0.4% for 3 days followed by 1-day preoperatively provided optimum efficacy and superior outcomes relative to 1 hour preoperatively used
Mathys et al. [48]	84	1. Nepafenac 0.01% (three times before surgery) + prednisolone acetate 1% 2. Nepafenac 0.01% (three times before surgery and for 1 month) + prednisolone acetate 1%	OCT 8 weeks	The increase in postoperative macular thickness was small in both the control and treatment groups
Miyake et al. [49]	80 eyes with primary open-angle glaucoma, normal tension glaucoma, or ocular hypertension	1. Fluorometholone acetate 2. 0.1% diclofenac sodium	FFA 5 weeks	Administration of nonsteroidal eye drops such as diclofenac seems to prevent macular edema formation enhanced by latanoprost therapy
Miyake et al. [50]	60 eyes with primary open-angle glaucoma, normal-tension glaucoma, or ocular hypertension	1. 0.1% fluorometholone acetate 2. 0.5% diclofenac sodium	FFA	Diclofenac prevents cystoid macular edema caused by timolol and its preservative, benzalkonium chloride
Miyanaga et al. [51]	72	1. 0.1% betamethasone 1 month, then 0.1% fluorometholone 1 month 2. 0.1% bromfenac for 2 months 3. 0.1% betamethasone 1 month, then 0.1% fluorometholone 1 month, and 0.1% bromfenac twice 2 months	OCT 2 months	There were no significant differences in anti-inflammatory effects among the three groups

Study	Number	Groups	Follow-up	Conclusion
Moschos et al. [52]	79	1. Dexamethasone sodium phosphate 0.1% 2. Dexamethasone sodium phosphate + diclofenac sodium 0.1%	OCT 28 days	The addition of diclofenac did not seem to offer any additional benefit after uneventful phacoemulsification
Ticly et al. [53]	91	1. Prednisolone acetate 1% 2. Prednisolone acetate 1% + ketorolac tromethamine 0.4%	FFA 5 weeks	The addition of ketorolac tromethamine 0.4% did not seem to offer any additional benefit after uneventful phacoemulsification
Wang et al. [54]	240	1. Oral prednisone tablets 15 mg for 7 days + fluorometholone 0.1% for 1 month 2. Oral prednisone tablets 15 mg for 7 days + dexamethasone 0.1% for 1 month 3. Oral prednisone tablets 15 mg for 7 days + bromfenac 0.1% for 1 month 4. Oral prednisone tablets 15 mg for 7 days + bromfenac 0.1% for 2 months	OCT 2 months	Bromfenac sodium was more effective and safer than fluorometholone and dexamethasone as an anti-inflammatory
Yavas et al. [55]	189	1. Prednisolone 2. Prednisolone + indomethacin for 3 days preoperative and 1 month postoperative 3. Prednisolone + indomethacin for 1 month postoperative	FFA 3 months	Preoperative nonsteroidal anti-inflammatory drugs decreased the incidence of CME more than postoperative use only
Capote et al. [56]	243	1. Diclofenac sodium 0.1% 2. Bromfenac 0.09% 3. Nepafenac 0.1% All received prednisolone 1%	OCT 6 months	Bromfenac is more effective than diclofenac and nepafenac in reducing macular thickness after phacoemulsification
McCafferty et al. [57]	1000	1. Placebo 2. Nepafenac 0.3%	OCT FFA 5 weeks	Topical nepafenac 0.3% reduces macular edema in patients with preoperative risk compared to placebo, but there were no differences in patients without risk factors
Stock et al. [58]	77	1. Nepafenac 2. Propylene glycol as control 3. Ketorolac tromethamine	OCT 45 days	There were no significant differences in macular thickness between the three groups

Study	Number	Groups	Follow-up	Conclusion
Milla et al. [59]	38 glaucoma patients	1. Nepafenac group (n = 15) 2. Nonnepafenac group (n = 23) All received dexamethasone	OCT	Nepafenac has a prophylactic effect aganist postoperative macular edema
Tzelikis et al. [60]	224	Bilateral cataract was included in this study Each patient was assigned randomly to receive nepafenac 0.3% drops in one eye and a placebo in the fellow eye	OCT 12 weeks	Nepafenac 0.3% was effective in reducing macular thickness compared with a placebo 5 weeks postoperatively

Table 4.
Clinical trials using ophthalmic NSAIDs to prevent postoperative macular edema in nondiabetic patients without cystoid macular edema preoperatively and with no predisposing factors for developing cystoid macular edema.

Donnenfeld et al. documented that early started ketorolac 3 days or 1 day preoperatively provided superior outcomes over ketorolac startes only 1 hour preoperatively [47]. Also, preoperative indomethacin drugs decreased the incidence of CME more than postoperative use only in the study of Yavas et al. [55].

In comparative study between different NSAIDs, Capote et al. approved that bromfenac is more effective than diclofenac and nepafenac in reducing macular thickness after phacoemulsification [56]. In other study, bromfenac was more effective and safer in comparison to topical steroid; inspite of using oral prednisones for all patients in the study [54].

In other studies, NSAIDs did not seem to offer any additional benefit after uneventful phacoemulsification of diclofenac in the study of Moschos et al. [52] and ketorolac in the study of Ticly et al. [53]. Miyanaga et al. documented that 2 months' use of topical NSAIDs, different topical steroids, or alternating steroids and NSAIDs had no significant differences [51]. Stock et al. suggested no differences between nepafenac, control, and ketorolac through 45-day follow-up [58].

Mathys et al. told that routine use of preoperative nepafenac may be necessary to achieve excellent visual recovery if continued for 3 weeks postoperatively or not [48].

In the study of McCafferty et al., postoperative topical nepafenac reduces macular edema in patients with preoperative risk (diabetic retinopathy, contralateral CME, or prostaglandin use) compared to placebo, but there were no differences in patients without risk factors [57]. Nepafenac was effective in reducing macular thickness compared with a placebo in fellow eye 5 weeks postoperatively in patients who had bilateral phacoemulsification enrolled in the study of Tzelikis et al. [60].

7. Conclusion(s)

The most important line of management of postoperative macular edema is by prevention. NSAIDs have large effects in prevention of postoperative macular edema with minimal side effects. Furthermore, some studies have suggested that NSAIDs may have a greater effect in re-establishment of the blood-aqueous barrier than corticosteroids. The claim about synergistic effects of NSAIDs and corticosteroids is made by several authors. Although several studies may have favored starting NSAID treatment preoperatively, there are no comparison studies about starting corticosteroids preoperatively.

Conflict of interest

The authors declare that they have no conflict of interest.

Author details

Ahmed Alnagdy[1*], Ahmed M. Eissa[2] and Amr El-Kannishy[1]

1 Mansoura Ophthalmology Center, Mansoura University, Egypt

2 The General Organization of Teaching Hospitals and Institutes, Egypt

*Address all correspondence to: alnagdy28@gmail.com

References

[1] DeBuc D, Somfai G. Early detection of retinal thickness changes in diabetes using optical coherence tomography. Medical Science Monitor. 2010;**16**: MT15-MT21

[2] Mentes J, Erakgun T, Afrashi F, Kerci G. Incidence of cystoid macular edema after uncomplicated phacoemulsification. Ophthalmologica. 2003;**217**:408-412. DOI: 10.1159/000073070

[3] Soliman W, Sander B, Jørgensen T. Enhanced optical coherence patterns of diabetic macular oedema and their correlation with the pathophysiology. Acta Ophthalmologica. 2007;**85**:613-617. DOI: 10.1111/j.1600-0420.2007.00917.x

[4] Lobo C. Pseudophakic cystoid macular edema. Ophthalmologica. 2012; **227**:61-67. DOI: 10.1159/000331277

[5] Miyake K, Ibaraki N. Prostaglandins and cystoid macular edema. Survey of Ophthalmology. 2002;**47**:S203-S218. DOI: 10.1016/S0039-6257(02)00294-1

[6] Krepler K, Biowski R, Schrey S, Jandrasits K, Wedrich A. Cataract surgery in patients with diabetic retinopathy: Visual outcome, progression of diabetic retinopathy, and incidence of diabetic macular oedema. Graefe's Archive for Clinical and Experimental Ophthalmology. 2002;**240**:735-738

[7] Schmier JK, Halpern MT, Covert DW, Matthews GP. Evaluation of costs for cystoid macular edema among patients after cataract surgery. Retina. 2007;**27**:621-628

[8] Sawides L, de Castro A, Burns S. The organization of the cone photoreceptor mosaic measured in the living human retina. Vision Research. 2016;**132**:34-44. DOI: 10.1016/j.visres.2016.06.006

[9] Spaide R, Klancnik J, Cooney M. Retinal vascular layers imaged by fluorescein angiography and optical coherence tomography angiography. JAMA Ophthalmology. 2015;**133**:45-50. DOI: 10.1001

[10] Ramírez J, Rojas B, Gallego B, García-Martín E, Triviño A, Ramírez A, et al. Glia and blood-retinal barrier: Effects of ocular hypertension. In: Cardiovascular Disease II. Hong Kong: Concept Press. 2014. pp. 123-162

[11] Cunha-Vaz J, Bernardes R, Lobo C. Blood-retinal barrier. European Journal of Ophthalmology. 2010;**21**:S3-S9. DOI: 10.1371/journal.pone.0095420

[12] Hori S, Ohtsuki S, Hosoya K, Nakashima E, Terasaki T. A pericyte-derived angiopoietin-1 multimeric complex induces occludin gene expression in brain capillary endothelial cells through tie-2 activation in vitro. Journal of Neurochemistry. 2004;**89**: 503-513. DOI: 10.1111/j.1471-4159.2004.02343.x

[13] Runkle E, Antonetti D. The blood-retinal barrier: Structure and functional significance. In: Nag S, The Blood-Brain and Other Neural Barriers: Reviews and Protocols. Totowa, NJ: Humana Press, Springer. 2011. pp. 133-148. https://doi.org/10.1007/978-1-60761-938-3_5

[14] Miyoshi J, Takai Y. Molecular perspective on tight-junction assembly and epithelial polarity. Advanced Drug Delivery Reviews. 2005;**57**:815-855. DOI: 10.1016/j.addr.2005.01.008

[15] Hee M, Izatt J, Swanson E, Huang D, Schuman J, Lin C, et al. Optical coherence tomography of the human retina. Archives of Ophthalmology. 1995;**113**:325-332. DOI: 10.1001/archopht.1995.01100030081025

[16] Gulkilik G, Kocabora S, Taskapili M, Engin G. Cystoid macular edema after phacoemulsification: Risk factors and

effect on visual acuity. Canadian Journal of Ophthalmology. 2006;**41**:699-703. DOI: 10.3129/i06-062

[17] Ursell P, Spalton D, Whitcup S, Nussenblatt R. Cystoid macular edema after phacoemulsification: Relationship to blood–aqueous barrier damage and visual acuity. Journal of Cataract and Refractive Surgery. 1999;**25**: 1492-1497. DOI: 10.1016/S0886-3350 (99)00196-0

[18] Kičová N, Bertelmann T, Irle S, Sekundo W, Mennel S. Evaluation of a posterior vitreous detachment: A comparison of biomicroscopy, B-scan ultrasonography and optical coherence tomography to surgical findings with chromodissection. Acta Ophthalmologica. 2012;**90**:e264-e268. DOI: 10.1111/j.1755-3768.2011.02330.x

[19] Vukicevic M, Gin T, Al-Qureshi S. Prevalence of optical coherence tomography-diagnosed postoperative cystoid macular oedema in patients following uncomplicated phaco-emulsification cataract surgery. Clinical & Experimental Ophthalmology. 2012; **40**:282-287. DOI: 10.1111/ j.1442-9071.2011.02638.x

[20] Muscat S, Parks S, Kemp E, Keating D. Repeatability and reproducibility of macular thickness measurements with the Humphrey OCT system. Investigative Ophthalmology & Visual Science. 2002;**43**:490-495

[21] Degenring R, Vey S, Kamppeter B, Budde W, Jonas J, Sauder G. Effect of uncomplicated phacoemulsification on the central retina in diabetic and non-diabetic subjects. Graefe's archive for. Clinical and Experimental Ophthalmology. 2007;**245**:18-23

[22] Cho H, Wolf K, Wolf E. Management of ocular inflammation and pain following cataract surgery: Focus on bromfenac ophthalmic solution. Clinical Ophthalmology. 2009; **3**:199-210

[23] Polansky J, Weinreb R. Anti-inflammatory agents. In: Pharmacology of the Eye. Berlin, Heidelberg: Springer; 1984. pp. 459-538. https://doi.org/ 10.1007/978-3-642-69222-2_11

[24] McGhee C, Dean S, Danesh-Meyer H. Locally administered ocular corticosteroids. Drug Safety. 2002;**25**: 33-55

[25] O'Brien T. Emerging guidelines for use of NSAID therapy to optimize cataract surgery patient care. Current Medical Research and Opinion. 2005;**21**: 1131-1137. DOI: 10.1185/ 030079905X50651

[26] Drugs@FDA [Internet]. 2018. Rockville (MD): Food and Drug Administration (US), Center for Drug Evaluation and Research. Available from: http://www.accessdata.fda.gov/scripts/cder/drugsatfda/index.cfm [cited: July 2018]

[27] Heier J, Topping T, Baumann W, Dirks M, Chern S. Ketorolac versus prednisolone versus combination therapy in the treatment of acute pseudophakic cystoid macular edema. Ophthalmology. 2000;**107**:2034-2038. DOI: 10.1016/S0161-6420(00)00365-1

[28] Alnagdy A, Abouelkheir H, El-Khouly S, Tarshouby S. Impact of topical nonsteroidal anti-inflammatory drugs in prevention of macular edema following cataract surgery in diabetic patients. International Journal of Ophthalmology. 2018;**11**(4):616-622. DOI: 10.18240/ijo.2018.04.133738

[29] Gaynes B, Fiscella R. Topical nonsteroidal anti-inflammatory drugs for ophthalmic use. Drug Safety. 2002; **25**:233-250

[30] Hernández-Díaz S, Rodríguez LAG. Association between nonsteroidal anti-

inflammatory drugs and upper gastrointestinal tract bleeding/perforation: An overview of epidemiologic studies published in the 1990s. Archives of Internal Medicine. 2000;**160**:2093-2099. DOI: 10.1001/archinte.160.14.2093

[31] Canto MG, Andreu I, Fernandez J, Blanca M. Selective immediate hypersensitivity reactions to NSAIDs. Current Opinion in Allergy and Clinical Immunology. 2009;**9**:293-297. DOI: 10.1097/ACI.0b013e32832db943

[32] Sun WH, Tsuji S, Tsujii M, Gunawan E, Sawaoka H, Kawai N, et al. Cyclo-oxygenase-2 inhibitors suppress epithelial cell kinetics and delay gastric wound healing in rats. Journal of Gastroenterology and Hepatology. 2000;**15**:752-761. DOI: 10.1046/j.1440-1746.2000.02242.x

[33] Sekhar C, Pathapati R, Varalakshmi U, Harshita S, Patra R, Divyalasya T. Head-to-head comparison of tolerability and acceptability of single dose of four topical NSAIDS in patients undergoing cataract surgery. Evidence-based Healthcare. 2015;**2**:4568-4573. DOI: 10.18410/jebmh/2015/643

[34] Endo N, Kato S, Haruyama K, Shoji M, Kitano S. Efficacy of bromfenac sodium ophthalmic solution in preventing cystoid macular oedema after cataract surgery in patients with diabetes. Acta Ophthalmologica. 2010; **88**(8):896-900. DOI: 10.1111/j.1755-3768.2009.01582.x

[35] Singh R, Alpern L, Jaffe G, et al. Evaluation of nepafenac in prevention of macular edema following cataract surgery in patients with diabetic retinopathy. Clinical Ophthalmology. 2012;**6**(1):1259-1269. DOI: 10.2147/OPTH.S31902. PMCID: PMC3422154

[36] Almeida D, Johnson D, Hollands H, et al. Effect of prophylactic nonsteroidal antiinflammatory drugs on cystoid macular edema assessed using optical coherence tomography quantification of total macular volume after cataract surgery. Journal of Cataract and Refractive Surgery. 2008;**34**(1):64-69. DOI: 10.1016/j.jcrs.2007.08.034

[37] Almeida D, Khan Z, Xing L, et al. Prophylactic nepafenac and ketorolac versus placebo in preventing postoperative macular edema after uneventful phacoemulsification. Journal of Cataract and Refractive Surgery. 2012;**38**(9):1537-1543. DOI: 10.1016/j.jcrs.2012.04.034

[38] Cable M. Comparison of bromfenac 0.09% QD to nepafenac 0.1% TID after cataract surgery: Pilot evaluation of visual acuity, macular volume, and retinal thickness at a single site. Clinical Ophthalmology. 2012;**6**(1):997-1004. DOI: 10.2147/OPTH.S32179. PMCID: PMC3399390

[39] Cervantes-Coste G, Sanchez-Castro YG, Orozco-Carroll M, Mendoza-Schuster E, Velasco-Barona C. Inhibition of surgically induced miosis and prevention of postoperative macular edema with nepafenac. Clinical Ophthalmology. 2009;**3**(1):219-226

[40] Rossetti L, Bujtar E, Castoldi D, Torrazza C, Orzalesi N. Effectiveness of diclofenac eyedrops in reducing inflammation and the incidence of cystoid macular edema after cataract surgery. Journal of Cataract and Refractive Surgery. 1996;**22**:794-799. DOI: 10.1016/S0886-3350(96)80164-7

[41] Miyake K, Masuda K, Shirato S, et al. Comparison of diclofenac and fluorometholone in preventing cystoid macular edema after small incision cataract surgery: A multicentered prospective trial. Japanese Journal of Ophthalmology. 2000;**44**(1):58-67. DOI: 10.1016/S0021-5155(99)00176-8

[42] Miyake K, Nishimura K, Harino S, et al. The effect of topical diclofenac on

choroidal blood flow in early postoperative pseudophakias with regard to cystoid macular edema formation. Investigative Ophthalmology & Visual Science. 2007;**48**(12): 5647-5652. DOI: 10.1167/iovs.07-0262

[43] Miyake K, Ota I, Miyake G, Numaga J. Nepafenac 0.1% versus fluorometholone 0.1% for preventing cystoid macular edema after cataract surgery. Journal of Cataract and Refractive Surgery. 2011;**37**(9): 1581-1588. DOI: 10.1167/iovs.07-0262

[44] Nishino M, Eguchi H, Iwata A, Shiota H, Tanaka M, Tanaka T. Are topical steroids essential after an uneventful cataract surgery? The Journal of Medical Investigation. 2009; **56**(1–2):11-15. DOI: 10.2152/jmi.56.11

[45] Weber M, Kodjikian L, Kruse F, Zagorski Z, Allaire C. Efficacy and safety of indomethacin 0.1% eye drops compared with ketorolac 0.5% eye drops in management of ocular inflammation after cataract surgery. Acta Ophthalmologica. 2013;**91**(1):e15-e21. DOI: 10.1111/j.1755-3768.2012.02520.x

[46] Wittpenn J, Silverstein S, Heier J, Kenyon K, Hunkeler J, Randomized EMA. Masked comparison of topical ketorolac 0.4% plus steroid vs steroid alone in low-risk cataract surgery patients. American Journal of Ophthalmology. 2008;**146**(4): 554-560. DOI: 10.1016/j.ajo.2008.04.036. e551

[47] Donnenfeld E, Perry H, Wittpenn J, Solomon R, Nattis A, Chou T. Preoperative ketorolac tromethamine 0.4% in phacoemulsification outcomes: Pharmacokinetic-response curve. Journal of Cataract and Refractive Surgery. 2006;**32**(9):1474-1482. DOI: 10.1016/j.jcrs.2006.04.009

[48] Mathys K, Cohen K. Impact of nepafenac 0.1% on macular thickness and postoperative visual acuity after cataract surgery in patients at low risk for cystoid macular oedema. Eye (London, England). 2010;**24**(1):90-96

[49] Miyake K, Ota I, Maekubo K, Ichihashi S, Miyake S. Latanoprost accelerates disruption of the blood-aqueous barrier and the incidence of angiographic cystoid macular edema in early postoperative pseudophakias. Archives of Ophthalmology. 1999; **117**(1):34-40. DOI: 10.1001/archopht.117.1.34

[50] Miyake K, Ota I, Ibaraki N, et al. Enhanced disruption of the blood-aqueous barrier and the incidence of angiographic cystoid macular edema by topical timolol and its preservative in early postoperative pseudophakia. Archives of Ophthalmology. 2001; **119**(3):387-394. DOI: :10.1001/archopht.119.3.387

[51] Miyanaga M, Miyai T, Nejima R, Maruyama Y, Miyata K, Kato S. Effect of bromfenac ophthalmic solution on ocular inflammation following cataract surgery. Acta Ophthalmologica. 2009; **87**(3):300-305. DOI: 10.1111/j.1755-3768.2008.01433.x

[52] Moschos M, Chatziralli I, Pantazis P, Rouvas A, Sergentanis T. Is topical diclofenac essential before and after uneventful phacoemulsification cataract surgery? Journal of Ocular Pharmacology and Therapeutics. 2012; **28**(4):335-339.29. DOI: 10.1089/jop.2011.0256

[53] Ticly F, Lira R, Zanetti F, Machado M, Rodrigues G, Arieta C. Prophylactic use of ketorolac tromethamine in cataract surgery: A randomized trial. Journal of Ocular Pharmacology and Therapeutics. 2014;**30**(6):495-501. DOI: 10.1089/jop.2013.0214

[54] Wang Q, Yao K, Xu W, et al. Bromfenac sodium 0.1%, fluorometholone 0.1% and

dexamethasone 0.1% for control of ocular inflammation and prevention of cystoid macular edema after phacoemulsification. Ophthalmologica. 2013;**229**(4):187-194. DOI: 10.1159/000346847

[55] Yavas G, Ozturk F, Kusbeci T. Preoperative topical indomethacin to prevent pseudophakic cystoid macular edema. Journal of Cataract and Refractive Surgery. 2007;**33**(5):804-807. DOI: 10.1016/j.jcrs.2007.01.033

[56] Capote A, Soto M, Ruiz R, Peláez C, Vazquez G, OftaCosta G, et al. Comparative study of the efficacy and safety of bromfenac, nepafenac and diclofenac sodium for the prevention of cystoid macular edema after phacoemulsification. International Journal of Ophthalmology. 2018;**11**(7):1210. DOI: 10.18240/ijo.2018.07.22

[57] McCafferty S, Harris A, Kew C, Kassm T, Lane L, Levine J, et al. Pseudophakic cystoid macular edema prevention and risk factors; prospective study with adjunctive once daily topical nepafenac 0.3% versus placebo. BMC Ophthalmology. 2017;**17**(1):16. DOI: 10.1186/s12886-017-0405-7

[58] Stock A, Galvan K, Godoy R, Bonamigo L. Comparison of macular thickness by optical coherence tomography measurements after uneventful phacoemulsification using ketorolac tromethamine, nepafenac, vs a control group, preoperatively and postoperatively. Clinical Ophthalmology. 2018;**12**:607. DOI: 10.2147/OPTH.S157738

[59] Milla E, Stirbu O, Franco J, Hernández G, Rios J, Duch S. Effect of nepafenac on the foveal profile of glaucomatous patients undergoing phacoemulsification. International Ophthalmology. 2017;**37**(5):1147-1153

[60] Tzelikis P, Morato C, Neves N, Hida W, Alves M. Intraindividual comparison of nepafenac 0.3% for the prevention of macular edema after phacoemulsification. Journal of Cataract & Refractive Surgery. 2018;**44**(4):440-446. DOI: 10.1016/j.jcrs.2018.01.026

Chapter 4

Prevalence and Association of Diabetic Retinopathy with Diabetic Foot Ulcer: A Cross-Sectional Observational Study

Shaista Zafar, Kashif Rahim, Inayat Ullah Khan, Muhammad Yasin, Muhammad Dawood and Shamim Saleha

Abstract

We aimed to elucidate prevalence and association of diabetic retinopathy (DR) in patients with diabetic foot ulcer (DFU) from Pakistan. In this cross-sectional study, about 225 DFU patients who underwent ophthalmic examinations within 6 months of diagnosis of foot ulceration were included. The medical records of 305 diabetic patients without DFU were included as controls. The association of DR with DFU was assessed by comparing DFU patients with proliferative DR (PDR) and DFU patients without PDR. Out of 225 DFU patients, 215 patients (95.6%) had DR and 169 patients (75.1%) had PDR. The prevalence of DFU was significantly greater ($P = 0.0527$) among the male diabetic patients, whereas advanced age of these patients (≥41 years) had a significant effect ($P = 0.0286$) on development and progression of PDR. A longer duration of diabetes (≥10 years) was identified as a significant contributing factor for the development of both DFU ($P = 0.0029$) and PDR ($P = 0.0299$). Moreover, the risk of PDR increased in diabetic patients with higher DFU grades (grade 3 and grade 4). In conclusion, retinopathy was prevalent in DFU patients. Therefore, DFU patients with advancing age and longer duration of diabetes should undergo retinal examinations for timely diagnosis and management of DR.

Keywords: diabetic foot ulcer, diabetic retinopathy, risk factors, Pakistan

1. Introduction

Diabetes mellitus (DM) is a metabolic disease, caused by chronic hyperglycemia as a result of defects in secretion of insulin, resistance to insulin action, or a combination of the two. Type 1 and type 2 are two main types of diabetes. Type 1 diabetes mellitus (T1DM) results from absolute deficiency of insulin secretion, and type 2 diabetes mellitus (T2DM) results from combined defects in both relative deficiency of insulin secretion and insulin resistance [1]. T2DM is the dominant form of diabetes which account to approximately >85% of all diabetes cases [2]. Diabetic foot ulcer (DFU) is the most devastating complication of diabetes, with a global prevalence of 6.3%, and is more common in patients with type 2 diabetes [3].

The lifetime risk of foot ulceration in patients with diabetes lies somewhere in the range of 15 and 25% [4, 5], with a yearly rate of around 2–3% [6].

Diabetic is associated with microvascular complications, including retinopathy, neuropathy, and nephropathy, and macrovascular complications, including ischemic coronary illness, stroke, and peripheral vascular disease [7]. Diabetic retinopathy (DR) is a common complication of diabetes that affects vision. DR damages the blood vessels of the light-sensitive tissue at the back of the eye (retina) that results in blindness if left undiagnosed and untreated. It is estimated that 20 years after diagnosis, those with type 1 diabetes and 60% of those with type 2 diabetes will have some level of retinopathy [8]. Approximately 4 million individuals around the globe are estimated to losing their sight from diabetic retinopathy, the main source of visual impairment in patients aged 20–74 years [9]. The risk of development and progression of DR is closely associated with the type 1 diabetes [8], longer duration of diabetes [10], advancing age [11], poor glycemic control [12], high blood pressure [13] and elevated serum lipids [14].

The descriptive analytical studies have demonstrated that diabetic retinopathy (DR) is among one of the major contributing factors in the development of foot ulceration and subsequent lower limb amputation in diabetic patients [11, 15–17]. Importantly, DFU patients with PAD are less likely to heal and more likely to require amputation compared to patients without PAD. Moreover, retinal screening in people with diabetic foot ulceration, followed by treatment of sight-threatening retinopathy, may prevent severe vision loss or blindness [18]. It is therefore essential that DR is diagnosed in all diabetic patients with a foot ulcer. There is a significant rise in the prevalence of diabetes and its complications in Pakistan, causing a major social and economic burden [19, 20]. Therefore, this study was conducted with an aim to investigate the prevalence of DR in patients with a DFU in Pakistan and to elucidate the potential association between DR and DFU.

2. Materials and methods

This was a cross-sectional observational study conducted in the diabetology clinic at Pakistan Institute of Medical Sciences (PIMS), located in federal capital of Pakistan, which is the largest tertiary care referral hospital. This study was conducted between March 2017 and February 2018 as per the guidelines of the Declaration of Helsinki, and the Institutional Ethical Committee approval was obtained before initiation. The study was explained, and written informed consent of the patients was obtained before their recruitment. Inclusion criteria were as follows: (1) all type 2 diabetic patients and only those type 1 diabetes patients with diabetes duration of more than 5 years, diagnosed with foot ulcers based on the Wagner ulcer classification, were included in this study. (2) Patients were included in the study only if they underwent ophthalmic examinations particularly funduscopy of the retina within 6 months after DFU diagnosis.

Participated DFU patients were classified into Wagner's grades [21] as follows: grade 1 (superficial ulcer), grade 2 (deep ulcer), grade 3 (ulcer with osteomyelitis), grade 4 (forefoot gangrene), and grade 5 (mid foot or hind foot gangrene). Moreover, the presence and severity of DR among DFU patients were assessed based on the grading of the Global Diabetic Retinopathy Project Group [22]. A five-stage disease severity classification for DR includes no apparent retinopathy (no DR), proliferative DR (PDR), and mild, moderate, or severe non-proliferative DR (NPDR). Clinical information and demographic details were obtained from medical records of participating patients. The medical records of diabetic patients without a DFU who also visited the diabetology clinic at PIMS for a health checkup were included as control.

Analysis of recruitment data was performed by using SPSS-PC version 16.0, and then tables and graphs were constructed to display characteristics of studied patients. The association between DR and DF was determined by using the Chi-square test. P-values <0.05 were considered significant.

3. Results

Data of patients recruited in the study was analyzed and summarized in **Table 1**. Among 225 patients with foot ulceration, majority of them were male (62.7%) and had type 2 (60%) diabetes. Most DFU patients were aged 41 years old and over (88.4%) and had diabetes since ≥10 years (65.8%), high HbA1c ≥ 7% (77.3%), and higher level of systolic blood pressure (72.4%). Statistically, significant differences were observed among diabetic patients with a foot ulcer or without a foot ulcer in relation to gender (P = 0.0527) and diabetes duration (P = 0.0029) only.

Additionally, DFU patients with PDR were compared with DFU patients without PDR as shown in **Table 1**. The PDR was less prevalent in diabetic males with foot ulcers (53.8%) in comparison to those without foot ulcers (66.1%). The DFU patients with PDR had type 2 diabetes (66.9%), advanced age (82.8%), longer

Characteristics of patients	Diabetes (N = 530)		P value	DFU (N = 225)		P value
	Diabetes with DFU (N = 225)	Diabetes without DFU (N = 305)		DFU with PDR (N = 169)	DFU without PDR (N = 56)	
Gender						
Male	141 (62.7)	215 (70.5)	0.0527*	91 (53.8)	37 (66.1)	0.1024
Female	84 (37.3)	90 (29.5)		78 (46.2)	19 (33.9)	
Age (years)						
≤41	26 (11.6)	37 (12.1)	0.7084	29 (17.2)	19 (33.9)	0.0286*
≥41	199 (88.4)	268 (87.9)		140 (82.8)	37 (66.1)	
Duration of diabetes (years)						
≤10	77 (34.2)	135 (44.3)	0.0029*	24 (14.2)	17 (30.4)	0.0299*
≥10	148 (65.8)	170 (55.7)		145 (85.8)	39 (69.6)	
Type of diabetes						
Type 1	90 (40)	111 (36.4)	0.3352	56 (33.1)	22 (39.3)	0.4170
Type 2	135 (60)	194 (63.6)		113 (66.9)	34 (60.7)	
HbA1c level						
≤ 7%	51 (22.7)	95 (31.1)	0.1638	30 (17.8)	11 (19.6)	0.7577
≥ 7%	174 (77.3)	210 (68.9)		139 (82.2)	45 (80.4)	
Blood pressure (mmHg)						
Systolic	163 (72.4)	229 (75.1)	0.4882	122 (72.2)	41 (73.2)	0.8807
Diastolic	62 (27.6)	76 (24.9)		47 (27.8)	15 (26.8)	

**Statistically significant*

Table 1.
Basic characteristics of diabetic patients with or without diabetic foot ulcer (DFU).

Types of DR	Diabetics with a DFU, N = 225(%)	Diabetics without a DFU, N = 305 (%)
No DR	10 (4.4)	255 (83.6)
Mild NPDR	11 (4.9)	10 (3.2)
Moderate NPDR	26 (11.6)	16 (5.2)
Severe NPDR	9 (4.0)	7 (2.3)
PDR	169 (75.1)	17 (5.6)

Table 2.
Prevalence of DR in patients with a DFU and in diabetic patients without a DFU .

duration of diabetes (85.8), high HbA1c ≥ 7% (82.2%), and elevated systolic blood pressure (72.2%) than DFU patients without PDR. The significant contributing factors of PDR among DFU patients were advanced age ($p = 0.0286$) and longer duration of diabetes (0.0299).

In terms of DR among diabetic patients with foot ulceration, 215 patients (95.6%) had DR and 169 patients (75.1%) had PDR. 11 patients (4.9%) had mild NPDR, 26 patients had moderate NPDR (11.6%), and 9 patients had severe NPDR (4.0%), as shown in **Table 2** and **Figure 1**. Moreover, the common ulcer grades were 3 (41.8%) and 4 (31.6%), among DFU patients with DR (**Table 3**).

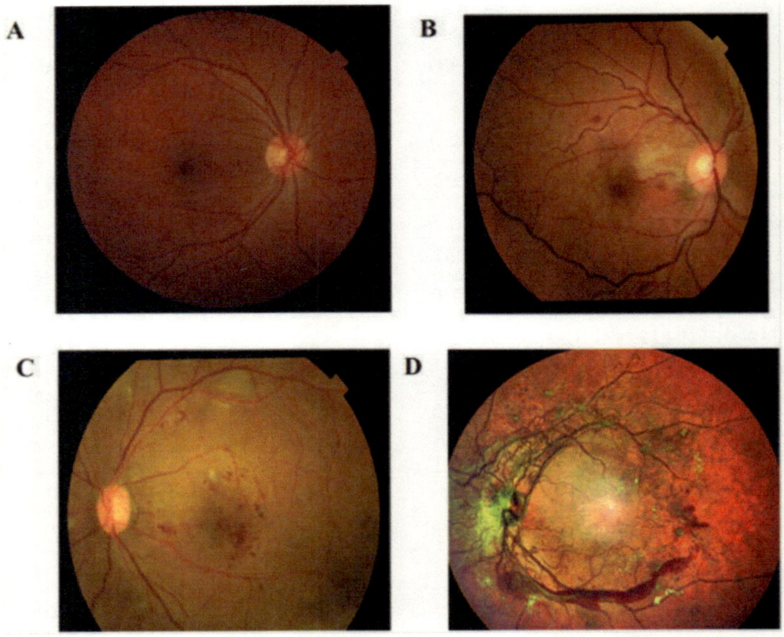

Figure 1.
Fundus photographs of some studied patients show clinical grades of DR. (A) Mild NPDR phenotypes based on the presence of only two microaneurysms and the absence of macular edema. (B) Moderate NPDR phenotypes based on the presence of scattered microaneurysms, dot-blot hemorrhages, hard exudates, and diffuse macular edema. (C) Severe NPDR phenotypes based on the presence of scattered microaneurysms, dot-blot hemorrhages, hard exudates, cotton wool spots, and clinically significant macular edema. (D) PDR phenotypes based on the presence of new vessels on the disc (NVD), new vessels elsewhere (NVE), preretinal hemorrhage, retinal hemorrhages, tractional bands, and laser marks of the previous pan retinal photocoagulation (PRP).

Wagner's grades	No DR, N = 10	Mild NPDR, N = 11	Moderate NPDR N = 26	Severe NPDR N = 9	PDR, N = 169	Total N (%)
Grade 1	2	1	3	0	17	23 (10.2)
Grade 2	1	3	3	2	28	37 (16.4)
Grade 3	4	5	11	2	72	94 (41.8)
Grade 4	3	2	9	5	52	71 (31.6)
Grade 5	0	0	0	0	0	0 (0)

Table 3.
Distribution of diabetic patients with DR according to ulcer grades.

4. Discussion

Diabetes is a common disease, associated with microvascular and macrovascular diseases that contribute to an increased risk of foot ulcers and subsequent lower extremity amputations in diabetic patients [7]. Population-based studies identified that DR is among one of the contributing diseases that significantly increased risk for foot ulceration in diabetic populations of Saudi Arabia [23], Korea [11], Spain [15], Iran [16] and India [17]. However, data is limited about contribution of DR in development of foot ulceration in diabetic population of Pakistan.

The present study revealed that the majority (95.7%) of DFU patients had DR, with 71.9% demonstrated PDR. A similar study reported that DR was prevalent (90%) in the US diabetic patients with foot ulcers, and about more than half of these patients had PDR [11]. Pemayun et al. in a hospital-based case-control study found PAD to be a major predictive factor for poor outcome among hospitalized DFU patients [24]. Previously, Nwanyanwu et al. in a retrospective cohort study assessed that chronic foot ulcers might contribute to retinopathy progression due to the reason that a significant proportion of diabetic chronic ulcer patients with NPDR who progressed to PDR in their analysis [25]. Among DFU patients with PDR, 73.4% had advanced Wagner's grades (grades 3 and 4) of foot ulceration in the present study. Hwang et al. found association of PDR with DFU and speculated that elevated oxidative stress and endothelial dysfunction can cause PDR in the advanced stages of diabetes [11].

The cross-sectional diabetes studies reported that prevalence of foot complications increases among diabetic males with advanced age and longer duration of diabetes [10, 11, 19, 23]. In the current study, diabetic patients with foot ulcers were compared with those without foot ulcers to find significant determinants for foot ulcer in diabetic patients, and it was found that a significant number of diabetic males were at a greater risk for the development of foot ulcers. Higher average height, higher plantar pressure, inadequate self-care practices, inappropriate shoes, and frequent exposure to traumatic events and frequently found peripheral insensate neuropathy have been identified as risk factors contributing to foot ulceration in diabetic males [26, 27]. Additionally, DFU patients were classified into the PDR or NPDR group; our results showed that diabetic males with foot ulcers had a higher prevalence of PDR comparatively to females, but this difference was not significant. Similarly, a diabetes study from the United Kingdom reported that PDR was more prevalent in males than in females [28]. In contrast, a community-based study in China showed that diabetic females were associated with increased risk of PDR [29]. This gender difference observed in present and previous studies could not identify it as a risk factor contributing to PDR in diabetic patients with foot ulceration.

Importantly, advancing age has been observed as a contributing factor to foot ulceration in diabetic patients in many studies [11, 23]. Although prevalence of foot ulcers was determined high among advanced age diabetic patients in current study, a statistically significant difference was not observed in terms of increasing age (≥41 years) of diabetic patients with and without foot ulceration. On the other hand, our study demonstrated statistically significant correlation between PDR and advanced age of DFU patients. In contrast to this observation, Hwang et al. [11] in a recent study failed to show a correlation between PDR and advanced age of DFU patients. Similarly, Li and Wang reported lower prevalence of DR in elderly diabetic patients and suggested that favorable control of blood glucose, blood pressure, and blood lipids effectively prevented the occurrence of DR in diabetic patients [30]. Therefore, it seems that high blood glucose levels and elevated systolic blood pressure have contributed to the developing of PDR in elderly DFU patients in current study.

Comparatively high prevalence of foot ulcers was observed among diabetic patients with diabetes duration more than 10 years in the current study, and this observation was significant. A previous study from Sudan supported our observation [10]. In two different previously conducted diabetic foot studies, the average duration of diabetes in DFU patients was 13.2 [31] and 8.2 years [32]. Based on current and previous observations, we hypothesize that the lengthy duration of diabetes is a significant risk factor for the development of diabetic foot ulceration. In addition, Chawla et al. in a study reported that chronic hyperglycemia and diabetes duration are among the main contributing factors to development and progression of DR in diabetic patients with foot ulcer [33]. The results of the present study also showed that lengthy duration of diabetes was a significant risk factor in progression of PDR among patients with DFU. In agreement with our results, Hwang et al. also reported that the foot ulcer patients with PDR had a longer duration of diabetes compared to those with NPDR [11].

5. Conclusion

In summary, the present study showed that a large proportion of advanced age patients with longer duration of diabetes had retinopathy and were at substantial risk of developing foot ulceration. Therefore, in advanced age DFU patients, and particularly those with longer duration of diabetes, early detection of DR and timely treatment may decrease the risk of severe vision loss or blindness.

Acknowledgements

This study was financially supported by the Department of Biotechnology and Genetic Engineering, Kohat University of Science and Technology. The authors acknowledge all those patients who participated in the study.

Conflict of interest

The author(s) declare that they have no competing interests.

Author details

Shaista Zafar[1], Kashif Rahim[2], Inayat Ullah Khan[1], Muhammad Yasin[3], Muhammad Dawood[3] and Shamim Saleha[3*]

1 Pakistan Institute of Medical Sciences (PIMS), Islamabad, Pakistan

2 Beijing Key Laboratory of Genetic Engineering Drug and Biotechnology, Institute of Biochemistry and Biotechnology, College of Life Sciences, Beijing Normal University, Beijing, China

3 Department of Biotechnology and Genetic Engineering, Kohat University of Science and Technology (KUST), Kohat, Khyber Pakhtunkhwa, Pakistan

*Address all correspondence to: shamimsaleha@yahoo.com

References

[1] Karalliedde J, Gnudi L. Diabetes mellitus, a complex and heterogeneous disease, and the role of insulin resistance as a determinant of diabetic kidney disease. Nephrology, Dialysis, Transplantation. 2016;**31**(2):206-213. DOI: 10.1093/ndt/gfu405

[2] Forouhi NG, Wareham NJ. Epidemiology of diabetes. Medicine (Abingdon). 2014;**42**(12):698-702. DOI: 10.1016/j.mpmed.2014.09.007

[3] Zhang et al. Global epidemiology of diabetic foot ulceration: A systematic review and meta-analysis. Annals of Medicine. 2017, 2017;**49**(2):106-116. DOI: 10.1080/07853890.2016.1231932

[4] Singh N, Armstrong DG, Lipsky BA. Preventing foot ulcers in patients with diabetes. Journal of the American Medical Association. 2005;**293**(2):217-228

[5] Wild S, Roglic G, Green A, Sicree R, King H. Global prevalence of diabetes: Estimates for the year 2000 and projections for 2030. Diabetes Care. 2004;**27**(5):1047-1053. DOI: 10.2337/diacare.27.5.1047

[6] Abbott CA, Carrington AL, Ashe H, Bath S, Every LC, Griffiths J, et al. The North-West Diabetes Foot Care Study: Incidence of, and risk factors for, new diabetic foot ulceration in a community-based patient cohort. Diabetic Medicine. 2002;**19**(5):377-384. DOI: 10.1046/j.1464-5491.2002.00698

[7] Orasanu G, Plutzky J. The pathologic continuum of diabetic vascular disease. Journal of the American College of Cardiology. 2009;**53**(5 Suppl):S35-S42. DOI: 10.1016/j.jacc.2008.09.055

[8] Watkins PJ. Retinopathy. BMJ. 2003;**326**(7395):924-926. DOI: 10.1136/bmj.326.7395.924

[9] Cheung N et al. Diabetic retinopathy. Lancet. 2010;**376**(9735):124-136. DOI: 10.1016/S0140-6736(09)62124-3

[10] Almobarak AO, Awadalla H, Osman M, Ahmed MH. Prevalence of diabetic foot ulceration and associated risk factors: An old and still major public health problem in Khartoum, Sudan? Annals of Translational Medicine. 2017;**5**(17):340. DOI: 10.21037/atm.2017.07.01

[11] Hwang DJ, Lee KM, Park MS, Choi SH, Park JI, Cho JH, et al. Association between diabetic foot ulcer and diabetic retinopathy. PLoS One. 2017;**12**(4):e0175270. DOI: 10.1371/journal.pone.0175270

[12] Fenwick EK, Xie J, Man REK, Sabanayagam C, Lim L, Rees G, et al. Combined poor diabetes control indicators are associated with higher risks of diabetic retinopathy and macular edema than poor glycemic control alone. PLoS One. 2017;**12**(6):e0180252. DOI: 10.1371/journal.pone.0180252

[13] Cardoso CRL, Leite NC, Dib E, Salles GF. Predictors of development and progression of retinopathy in patients with type 2 diabetes: Importance of blood pressure parameters. Scientific Reports. 2017;**7**(1):4867. DOI: 10.1038/s41598-017-05159-6

[14] Agroiya P, Philip R, Saran S, Gutch M, Tyagi R, Gupta KK. Association of serum lipids with diabetic retinopathy in type 2 diabetes. Indian Journal of Endocrinology and Metabolism. 2013;**17**(Suppl 1):S335-S337. DOI: 10.4103/2230-8210.119637

[15] Dòria M, Rosado V, Pacheco LR, Hernández M, Betriu À, Valls J, et al. Prevalence of diabetic foot disease in patients with diabetes

under renal replacement tin Lleida, Spain. BioMed Research International. 2016;**2016**:7217586. DOI: 10.1155/2016/7217586

[16] Maroufizadeh S, Almasi-Hashiani A, Hosseini M, Sepidarkish M, Omani Samani R. Prevalence of diabetic retinopathy in Iran: A systematic review and meta-analysis. International Journal of Ophthalmology. 2017;**10**(5):782-789. DOI: 10.18240/ijo.2017.05.21

[17] Karam T, Kamath YS, Rao LG, Rao KA, Shenoy SB, Bhandary SV. Diabetic retinopathy in patients with diabetic foot syndrome in South India. Indian Journal of Ophthalmology. 2018;**66**(4):547-550. DOI: 10.4103/ijo.IJO_1000_17

[18] Brownrigg JR, Apelqvist J, Bakker K, Schaper NC, Hinchliffe RJ. Evidence-based management of PAD & the diabetic foot. European Journal of Vascular and Endovascular Surgery. 2013;**45**(6):673-681. DOI: 10.1016/j.ejvs.2013.02.014

[19] Shera AS, Jawad F, Maqsood A. Prevalence of diabetes in Pakistan. Diabetes Research and Clinical Practice. 2007;**76**(2):219-222. DOI: 10.1016/j.diabres.2006.08.011

[20] Basit A, Fawwad A, Qureshi H, Shera AS, NDSP Members. Prevalence of diabetes, pre-diabetes and associated risk factors: Second National Diabetes Survey of Pakistan (NDSP), 2016-2017. BMJ Open. 2018 5;**8**(8):e020961. DOI: 10.1136/bmjopen-2017-020961

[21] Lipsky BA, Berendt AR, Deery HG, Embil JM, Joseph WS, Karchmer AW, et al. Diagnosis and treatment of diabetic foot infections. Plastic and Reconstructive Surgery. 2006;**117**(7 supplement):212S-238S. DOI: 10.1097/01.prs.0000222737.09322.77

[22] Wilkinson CP, Ferris FL 3rd, Klein RE, Lee PP, Agardh CD, Davis M, et al. Proposed international clinical diabetic retinopathy and diabetic macular edema disease severity scales. Ophthalmology. 2003;**110**(9):1677-1682. DOI: 10.1016/S0161-6420(03)00475-5

[23] Al-Rubeaan K, Al Derwish M, Ouizi S, Youssef AM, Subhani SN, Ibrahim HM, et al. Diabetic foot complications and their risk factors from a large retrospective cohort study. PLoS One. 2015;**10**(5):e0124446. DOI: 10.1371/journal.pone.0124446

[24] Pemayun TGD, Naibaho RM, Novitasari D, et al. Risk factors for lower extremity amputation in patients with diabetic foot ulcers: A hospital-based case-control study. Diabetic Foot Ankle. 2015;**6**:29629. DOI: 10.3402/dfa.v6.29629

[25] Harris Nwanyanwu K, Talwar N, Gardner TW, Wrobel JS, Herman WH, Stein JD. Predicting development of proliferative diabetic retinopathy. Diabetes Care. 2013;**36**(6):1562-1568. DOI: 10.2337/dc12-0790

[26] Al-Mahroos F, Al-Roomi K. Diabetic neuropathy, foot ulceration, peripheral vascular disease and potential risk factors among patients with diabetes in Bahrain: A nationwide primary care diabetes clinic-based study. Annals of Saudi Medicine. 2007;**27**(1):25-31. DOI: 10.4103/0256-4947.51536

[27] Peek ME. Gender differences in diabetes-related lower extremity amputations. Clinical Orthopaedics and Related Research. 2011;**469**(7):1951-1955. DOI: 10.1007/s11999-010-1735-4

[28] Kohner EM, Aldington SJ, Stratton IM, Manley SE, Holman RR, Matthews DR, et al. United Kingdom Prospective Diabetes Study, 30: Diabetic retinopathy at diagnosis of non-insulin-dependent diabetes mellitus and associated risk factors. Archives of Ophthalmology. 1998;**116**(3):297-303. DOI: 10.1001/archopht.116.3.297

[29] Wang J, Zhang RY, Chen RP, Sun J, Yang R, Ke XY, et al. Prevalence and risk factors for diabetic retinopathy in a high-risk Chinese population. BMC Public Health. 2013;**13**:633. DOI: 10.1186/1471-2458-13-633

[30] Li X, Wang Z. Prevalence and incidence of retinopathy in elderly diabetic patients receiving early diagnosis and treatment. Experimental and Therapeutic Medicine. 2013;**5**(5):1393-1396. DOI: 10.3892/etm.2013.1021

[31] Boyko EJ, Ahroni JH, Stensel V, Forsberg RC, Davignon DR, Smith DG. A prospective study of risk factors for diabetic foot ulcer. The Seattle Diabetic Foot Study. Diabetes Care. 1999;**22**:1036-1042. DOI: 10.2337/diacare.22.7.1036

[32] Chalya PL, Mabula JB, Dass RM, Kabangila R, Jaka H, McHembe MD, et al. Surgical management of Diabetic foot ulcers: A Tanzanian University Teaching Hospital experience. BMC Research Notes. 2011;**4**:365. DOI: 10.1186/1756-0500-4-365

[33] Chawla A, Chawla R, Jaggi S. Microvascular and macrovascular complications in diabetes mellitus: Distinct or continuum? Indian Journal of Endocrinology and Metabolism. 2016;**20**(4):546-551. DOI: 10.4103/2230-8210.183480

Chapter 5

Clinical Evaluation of Horizontal Pediatric Strabismus and the Management Challenges

Lawan Abdu

Abstract

Pediatric strabismus is not uncommon. Poor knowledge and religious and cultural practices result in inattention to the child's need and stigmatization. Horizontal strabismus consisting of esotropia and exotropia constitutes the common types presenting. Childhood ocular deviations are associated with uncorrected refractive errors, diseases causing obstruction of the visual axis such as cataract, and intra ocular tumors commonly retinoblastoma. In parts of the developing world, there is poor documentation and recollection of medical events at family and community levels. Squint in a child is not a painful dramatic condition that can prompt quick action from the parents or caregiver. There is generalized inequity in access to health care. Pediatric ophthalmic services are at best in developmental stage, and purpose design service centers are quite few. Neglect of the causes and timely treatment of amblyopia can retard child's development resulting in dependency and aggravation of poverty circle. A comprehensive approach to management of childhood eye diseases including strabismus is desirable in the low income developing countries. Provision of health insurance as a citizen's right will reduce most of the health challenges.

Keywords: horizontal, strabismus, challenges, management, low income

1. Introduction

Strabismus is defined as deviation from normal position of alignment resulting in the eyes pointing in different directions [1]. From the historical perspective existed, the concept that there is spasm of the bodies which move the eye balls and there is oblique tendency of the muscles [2]. Ocular movement is controlled by six muscles comprising the four recti muscles (superior, inferior, medial, and lateral) which arises from the annulus of Zinn [3]—a fibrous structure which is fused to the optic nerve and foramen and the two oblique muscles [4]. The medial rectus takes a course close to the medial orbital wall, while the lateral rectus course is close to the lateral orbital wall before they reach their respective points of insertion. Primary action of medial rectus is adduction and lateral rectus abduction. The two are called the horizontal recti muscles. The superior and inferior recti muscles are called vertical muscles. The superior rectus muscle ran a course anteriorly above the eye ball, over the insertion of the superior oblique forming an angle of 23° with the visual axis. The primary function of superior rectus is elevation, secondary action is intorsion, and tertiary action is abduction. The inferior rectus passes anteriorly above the orbital floor and below the eye ball to which it is inserted at 23° to the visual axis. In the primary position, the main action of inferior rectus is depression, secondary action is extortion, and tertiary action is adduction. Superior oblique arises from the orbital apex above the annulus of Zinn, courses anteriorly close to the superior medial orbital wall. It becomes tendinous as it passes through the trochlear—a cartilage-like structure attached to the superior nasal orbital part of the frontal bone. The muscle tendon turns backward and inserted in the posterior medial quadrant of the eye ball under the superior rectus muscle forming a 51° angle with the visual axis [5]. In primary position, the action of superior oblique is intorsion, secondary action is depression, and tertiary action is abduction. Inferior oblique muscle originates from the periosteum of the maxillary bone behind the orbital rim and lateral to the entrance of the lacrimal fossa. It then passes laterally, superiorly, and posteriorly below the inferior rectus, under the lateral rectus and inserted into the posterior lateral quadrant of the eye ball. In the primary position, its primary action is extortion, secondary action is elevation, and tertiary action is abduction. The spiral of Tillaux describes the distance in millimeters from limbus to the insertion point of the four recti muscle: superior rectus (7.7 mm), lateral (96.9 mm), inferior (6.5 mm), and medial (5.5 mm). The lateral rectus is supplied by the abducent nerve, superior oblique by trochlear nerve, and the oculomotor nerve supplies all the rest (superior/medial/inferior recti and inferior oblique). Extra ocular muscles are supplied by muscular branches of the ophthalmic artery. The larger medial muscular branch supplies the inferior/medial recti and inferior oblique, while the lateral muscular branch supplies the lateral/superior recti, superior oblique, and the levator palpebrae superioris muscle. Eye movements can be uniocular (ductions) or binocular (versions). Movement of the eye nasally is called adduction, temporally abduction, downward infraduction, and upward supraduction. Nasal rotation of the superior corneal meridian is called intorsion or incycloduction, while temporal rotation is termed extortion or excycloduction. An agonist is the primary muscle involved in moving the eye in a given direction. A synergist is the muscle in the same eye that acts with the agonist to produce a given movement. An antagonist is a muscle in the same eye that produces action opposite that of the agonist. According to Sherrington's law [6] of reciprocal innervation, increased innervation and contraction of a given extra ocular muscle is associated with decrease innervation and contraction of its antagonist. Conjugate binocular eye movements which ensure the eyes move in the same direction are called versions; disconjugate movements which make the eyes move in opposite directions are called vergences. By this notation, right gaze is dextroversion, left levoversion, upward sursumversion, and downward deorsumversion. Rotating the eyes such that such that the superior pole of both corneal meridians is turned to the right is called dextrocycloversion, when to the left levocycloversion. Yoke muscles are two muscles in separate eyes that are prime movers for any given position [7]. All the muscles have respective partners that they work simultaneously to produce binocular movement. According to Hering's law [8] of motor correspondence, equal and simultaneous innervation goes to yoke muscles to produce binocular movement in desired direction. Convergence arises when the two eyes move nasally from any initial position, and divergence is when they move temporally from relative initial position. Nasal rotation of the vertical pole of both corneal meridians is incyclovergence, while temporal rotation is excyclovergence. The relative position of the eyes at rest is that of divergence, hence tonic convergence maintains the position of the eyes during wake period. The synkinetic near reflex consists of accommodation, convergence, and miosis. There is consistent increase in accommodative convergence (AC) for each diopter of accommodation (A) [9]. When the accommodative convergence/accommodation (AC/A) ratio is high, excess convergence could result in esotropia when viewing near objects. Voluntary convergence can consciously be induced as part of the near synkinesis. Proximal convergence can be produced based on the psychological awareness of nearness of the object. Bitemporal retinal image disparity stimulates fusional convergence which insures the image of an object is projected on corresponding retinal points. Conversely, fusional divergence could occur as an optomotor reflex to align the eyes so that images fall on corresponding retinal points. Retina stimulation is perceived as light coming from a specific visual direction in space. Retinal correspondence is said to occur when light stimulates two points in both eyes which share a common visual direction. Corresponding retinal points share a common relationship with the fovea in both eyes, and such relationship is described as normal retinal correspondence (NRC) [10]. Anomalous retinal correspondence (ARC) occurs when two points in the retina of both eyes do not share similar relationship with the fovea. Normal fovea and extra foveal NRC result in binocular single vision. Similarly, points in both eyes with similar fixation/orientation appear singly so far as they fall on a point that passes through the optical center of each eye and fixation point (Vieth-Muller circle). The process of cortical image unification of objects that fall on corresponding retinal points is called fusion. Retinal images are fused in the cortex when they are similar in shape, size, and clarity. Fusion has sensory, motor, and stereopsis components. The sensory part deals with relationship of the retinal points in the two eyes, while motor fusion is vergence movement that ensures retinal image fall and is maintained on corresponding points. Stereopsis is said to occur when disparity in image size is big enough not to permit cortical fusion but not enough to cause diplopia. Stereopsis is a binocular perception of depth that adds to quality of vision and three dimensions.

2. Visual assessment in children

The techniques of assessing vision in children are tailored to fit the patient's age. It is often challenging and tasking irrespective of the age and requires gaining the trust of the child and the parent. The clinic environment should to some extent fit ideal setting to do so. This is frequently not available in some low income countries as few pediatric ophthalmic clinics are purposefully designed. Frequently, the same make soft clinic area is used for all purposes. The CSM (Central, Steady, and Maintained) criterion can be used for preverbal children. This involves determining the location of the corneal reflex which should be central in a normal child while mono-fixating with the contra lateral eye occluded. The location of the reflex should be central in both eyes as uncentral position is abnormal. The fixation should be steadily (S) maintained with the light in stationary position and when moved in other directions. Fixation should be (M) maintained in both eyes, and failure in one eye may indicate the presence of amblyopia. A child would elicit avoidance movement when the seeing eye is occluded and can be indifferent when occlusion involves an amblyopic eye. Illiterate "E" chart "game" can be used to assess vision in preschool children. HOTV test can be used as it employs matching of objects placed on the distant display and a hand held version that enables the child to indicate similar images. Children of school age can have vision tested with Snellen's chart which has the drawback of crowding of letters that make its use limited in those with amblyopia. Various picture charts are developed showing objects that are commonly seen in the locality instead of trains and busses that may be unfamiliar to children in the developing world.

2.1 Light reflex test

Light reflex tests consist of the Hirschberg and Karimsky. The Hirschberg test measures the extent of decentration of the corneal reflex, and 1 mm of decentration is equivalent to 7° or 15 prism diopters. When the light reflex is at pupillary margin, there is (15°), mid iris is (30°), and at limbus (45°) of deviation, respectively. The Krimsky test uses corneal reflex from both eyes and a prism is placed before the fixating eye and adjusted till alignment is achieved. The test is ideally performed at near gaze position. To a lesser extent, Bruckner's test [11] can be used to detect (without quantifying) the presence of a squint. Light from an ophthalmoscope is shone directly into both eyes, and the reflection from the deviating eye is brighter than in the fixating eye. The light reflex tests can be affected by angle kappa (the angle between the anatomical and visual axis of the eye). In normal situations, the fovea is usually temporal to the pupillary center making the corneal reflex slightly nasal (the resulting positive angle Kappa that appears like an exodeviation), and this can affect the light reflex test though it has no impact on cover tests.

2.2 Cover tests

Cover tests are employed to assess misalignment. Monoocular test such as cover-uncover is used to distinguish heterophoria from heterotropia. When one eye is covered, the uncovered eye moves to take up aligned position, and the movement is reversed when the cover is removed. The test is based on the principle that breaking up of binocular vision during the test leads to adjustment in alignment in those with phorias. In the presence of manifest squint, the test is started with a deviated eye, and at the end, it is noted that the deviation is maintained by the index or contra lateral eye. Alternate cover test is done to determine and quantify the extent of deviation whether latent or manifest by the placement of a prism is in front of the eye. The base of the prism is placed opposite the direction of the deviation. The amount of deviation is measured with prisms as the cover is moved from one eye to another till alignment is achieved. Simultaneous prism and cover test can be employed to determine extend of manifest deviation when both eyes are uncovered [12].

2.3 Dissimilar image test

Dissimilar image tests involve making the images appear dissimilar in both eyes. The principle is that in the normal eye, the image falls on the fovea, while in the deviating eye, it falls elsewhere in the retina. A patient sees the images appearing somewhat homonymously in esotropia and crossed in exotropia. The Maddox rod consists of parallel cylinders that convert a point source of light into a straight line that is at right angle to the arranged cylinders. In normal situation of orthophoria, a person looking at a distant pointed light source with the rod placed before one eye would see a straight line (with the eye wearing the Maddox rod) and a point source of light (with the other eye). The light spot will appear to be at the center of the line. Maddox rod can be used to measure horizontal and vertical deviations. The relationship of the line relative to the spot of light determines the type of deviation. To quantify the deviation, a prism can be placed before the deviating eye till the state or orthophoria is achieved with the spot of light superimposed on the middle of the line. Cyclo deviations can also be measured with double Maddox road [13].

2.4 Dissimilar target test

This test involves making the eyes to be exposed to different targets at the same time and measuring the extent of deviation with one eye fixating then the other. Patients with esotropia will have crossed fixation and exotropes homonymous diplopia. The Lancaster red-green test consists of red-green goggles that can be reversed, red/green slit projector, and a ruled screen with many small squares. With red lens on the right, the patient is requested to superimpose the green slit, and the goggles are reversed to run the test again. This test is done in patients with diplopia from incomitant squint and may not apply to children who rarely present with this type. The mayor amblyoscope is calibrated to measure the extent of vertical, horizontal, and torsional deviations when the patient look through and superimpose dissimilar targets.

2.5 Historical perspective

Children require an adult who may be a parent, sibling, or other relations to accompany them to the hospital. The mother is the person closest to the child and in better position to offer more reliable information on the ocular condition of the patient. However due to religious and socio cultural practices, it is not unusual to see grandmothers and other relations who have minimal knowledge are made to accompany the children to the clinic. In vast rural communities, there is virtually no documentation of medical illness and recollection of what happens in the past is quite vague. Coverage of antenatal care by orthodox methods is largely poor with cost, distance, and attitude of healthcare providers constituting a barrier. Squint and other ocular conditions that are not associated with dramatic pain or debility may not attract attention warranting prompt medical care. There is varied individual and community perception of squint based on cultural and religious beliefs resulting in poor awareness of the cause and availability of treatment often leading to social stigmatization [14]. There is poor perception of strabismus in community that could partly be due to poor knowledge of the condition [15]. Deviating eye may be considered as an act of creation by God. In some communities, there is taboo and superstition attached to it resulting in stigmatization and ostracism. In the United States, an estimated 4% of children have strabismus [1]. In sub-Saharan Africa, population prevalence statistics are at best scarce, and the exact extent is likely to be known. A study involving thousands of elementary school children showed that esotropia and exotropia occurred in 0.14% of the population [16]. The prevalence varies between countries and the type of study conducted ranging from 0 to 2% in Ghana [17], 1.1% in Ethiopia [18], 0.5% in Tanzania [19], and 1.22% in Cameroons [20]. As much as is realizable, it is important to determine the onset, description of the type, laterality, variation with time, and duration of the deviation. Key knowledge includes determining whether it affects one eye or alternates. Any associated ocular features such as leucocoria to suggest secondary causes like cataract and retinoblastoma [21]. The clinician should obtain the history of previous spectacle prescriptions or ocular surgery performed. There may be a positive family history of similar symptoms and where available photographs could provide further clues in the patient's evaluation.

2.6 Definition and classification

Strabismus is a Greek term which simply means ocular misalignment. Manifest deviations that are detectable when both eyes are opened are called tropia and may present as a constant or intermittent deviation involving one eye or both eyes. Latent deviations are termed phorias and detectable only when one eye is covered so that the vision is monocular. In phorias, the misalignment is minor and corrected by cortical adjustment of the extra ocular muscles. Deviations are said to be comitant when they are the same in amplitude and degree of misalignment in all directions of gaze. Incomitant deviations vary in degree and amplitude with direction of gaze. Horizontal deviations could be nasal termed as esotropia or temporal exotropia. Other less common deviations in childhood include vertical (hyper deviation or hypo deviation) and torsional (incyclodeviation or excyclodeviation). Deviation could also manifest as a combination of the above. Pediatric strabismus can be infantile or acquired. Risk factors for infantile strabismus include a positive family history among first and second degree relatives, maternal alcohol ingestion in pregnancy, maternal smoking [22], genetic disorders (such as Crouzon's and Down's syndromes), prematurity and or, low birth weight, congenital ocular defects, and cerebral palsy. Causes of acquired strabismus include refractive error (particularly hyperopia), head injury that could include birth trauma, and neurological conditions (such as cranial nerve palsy involving nerves 3, 4, 6, and spina bifida).

2.7 Infantile esotropia

Esodeviations can be described as a latent or manifest convergent ocular misalignment. The latent type (esophoria) is negated by the fusional mechanism of the brain. Intermittent esotropia is the type that is to some extent controlled by fusional mechanism, and deviations manifest under conditions of stress or fatigue when the fusional mechanism becomes obviated. Esotropia noted within the first 6 months of life is termed infantile (or congenital) and in most instances is present in an otherwise normal child. Although the etiology is unclear, Worth's concept postulates a deficiency in cortical in the brain, while Chavasse postulates a possible mechanical cause [23], and thus cure can be achieved by eliminating the deviation in infancy. In developed countries where health documentation is the norm, a positive family is often present, while in sub Saharan Africa, such information is rarely obtained. Children with esotropia elicit alternate fixation, those with large angle deviation uses the adducted eye to fixate on objects in the contra lateral visual field (crossed fixation). The deviation is large and often greater than 30 prism diopters. Quite frequently the patients tend to have demonstrable inferior oblique overreaction in over 50% [24].

2.7.1 Management of infantile esotropia

The assessment of degree and extend of deviation are important in addition to cycloplegic fundal examination to rule out other secondary causes of misalignment such as a cataract or retinoblastoma. There may be a need to examine and refract the child under anesthesia. This warrants clinical examination by a pediatrician in addition to laboratory tests such as electrolytes and urea, and hemogram and hemoglobin electrophoresis as sickle cell disorder is frequent in SSA. Cycloplegic refraction often reveals a hyperopia of not more than two diopters, though in some instances, patients may be myopic or have astigmatism. It is necessary to correct any detected refractive error fully and promptly. In most instances, surgical correction is required preferably within the first 24 months of life. Early surgery is aimed at reducing deviation as much as could be achieved and obtaining orthotropia. This would enable better alignment and achieving fusion [25], characterized by favorable cosmetic appearance, improved peripheral fusion, and central suppression.

2.8 Acquired esotropia

This includes accommodative [26], nonaccommodative, and nystagmus associated esotropia. Accommodative esotropia presents between second and third year of life and is associated with activation of the accommodation reflex. It is characteristically intermittent at onset and later becomes constant and there may be associated amblyopia. In aged children, diplopia may be elicited before the onset of facultative suppressive scotoma. This type of esotropia has a hereditary component and could be precipitated by illness or trauma. Refractive accommodative esotropia is associated with hypermetropia, accommodative convergence, and insufficient fusional divergence. The esotropia is equal for both far and near fixation. Treatment involves cycloplegic refraction and dispensing of full correction to ensure good outcome [27]. Parental counseling to ensure constant use of spectacle correction is important in achieving compliance. Children who manifest non-accommodative component or fail to regain fusion with glasses may require surgery.

2.9 Accommodative esotropia

The accommodative synkinetic reflex consists of accommodative esotropia, convergence, and miosis. The age of onset range ages between 6 months and 7 years; it is intermittent at onset, and later becomes constant; symptoms may be precipitated by trauma or illness; and often there is associated amblyopia and is of hereditary nature.

2.10 Refractive accommodative esotropia

This type of esotropia is associated with uncorrected hyperopia, accommodative convergence, and fusional divergence insufficiency. Accommodation is stimulated due to existing hyperopia to obtain better retinal focus. Accommodative esotropia accounted for 18% of 7000 school children is examined [16]. Esotropia could manifest early [28], and the extent of deviation is the same for far and near. The amount of hyperopia is about +4 diopters, and the degree of deviation is in the range of 30–40 prism diopters. The aim is to do a cycloplegic refraction and offer full correction to be worn at all times. Counseling of the parents is important as treatment may not completely eliminate the deviation. Indication for surgical correction includes failure to attain fusion and presence of nonaccommodative component of the deviation.

2.11 Esotropia with high accommodative convergence/accommodative ratio

This type of esotropia can be refractive or nonrefractive. In hyperopia, excess convergence can result with accommodation for near objects. The degree of esotropia is more for near than distance vision. There is a detectable difference in extent with varied distance of accommodation. Nonrefractive accommodative esotropia can occur with normal levels of hyperopia, astigmatism, and myopia. Refractive esotropia with high AC/A can occur with hyperopia, and when associated with myopia or emmetropia, it is described as nonrefractive accommodative esotropia. Partially, accommodative esotropia could arise from decompensation of fully accommodative esotropia or an esotropia that develop subsequent accommodative component.

2.12 Management of esotropia with high AC/A

Bifocals are prescribed for treatment of nonrefractive accommodative esotropia. Flat top executive types of bifocal are preferred with power of +3.00 diopter sphere. The caregiver needs to be advised on consistent use and patient monitored to achieve restoration of fusion and stereopsis. The goal is to attain fusion with less than 10 prism diopters of residual esotropia for near vision with patient wearing the correction. Relative high AC/A has been observed even with bifocals use over time period [29]. Other measures include use of long-acting anticholinesterases such as 0.125% ecothiopate iodide drops. The treatment should commence with maximum dose and tailored based on response. Anticholinesterases have complications arising from depletion of pseudocholinesterases leading to increased susceptibility to depolarizing muscle blockers such as succinylcholine. Surgery can be performed to correct the esotropia instead of the earlier listed modalities. The normal trend with hyperopia is that it increases about the age of 5–7 years. Partially, accommodative esotropia is treated with full cycloplegic refraction and prescription of full correction. There is often a need for concurrent treatment of associated amblyopia.

2.13 Nonaccommodative acquired esotropia

This type of esotropia presents between the ages of 1 and 5 years. It may acutely present the following disruption of binocular vision from amblyopia treatment or after ocular injury. There may be associated underlying neurological disease or malignancy [30]. When clinical neurological assessment is normal, binocular vision is restored with prisms or surgery.

2.14 Sensory deprivation esotropia

This arises from occlusion of the visual axis from other ocular condition such as cataract [31], corneal opacity, glaucoma [32], and retinoblastoma [21]. This requires prompt removal of the underline cause wherever possible and treatment of any resulting amblyopia.

2.15 Surgical esotropia

Surgical esotropia is also referred to as consecutive esotropia. This form of esotropia arises as a result of surgical correction of exotropia (perhaps due to overcorrection). The deviation may improve spontaneously and when it this doesn't happen, prisms are used to correct it. The presence of abduction deficiency should raise suspicion of a slipped lateral rectus muscle [33], and patient may require transposition procedure.

2.16 Near synkinetic reflex spasm

The near reflex has accommodative, convergence, and miosis components. There may be a manifest cycle of esotropia and orthotropia. The cause may not necessarily be organic and could be due to psychological factors. The patient has no demonstrable abduction paralysis. Cycloplegic refraction and prompt correction lead to improvement, and in the presence of hyperopia, the patient may require bifocal correction.

2.17 Incomitant esotropia

This deviation varies in severity with the position of gaze and is due to abducent nerve paralysis. Cross fixation can be mistaken for this type of esotropia. In the absence of strabismic amblyopia, the vision in both eyes is comparably normal. Sixth nerve paralysis is rare at infancy, and its presence in childhood should raise the suspicion of an intracranial mass. Therefore, full neurological screening including brain CT scan and MRI is needed. Infectious causes such as meningococcal and tuberculous meningitis are more common causes in SSA. Treatment involves correction of any associated hyperopia, patch therapy for amblyopia, and use of membrane (Fresnel-press on) prism. Those with underlying medical condition should be treated in collaboration with respective specialists.

2.18 Exotropia

Divergent squints can be latent (exophoria-negated by the fusional mechanism) or manifest (exotropia). Exophorias can be demonstrated by breaking the fusional mechanism (uniocular occlusion as in cover test). Exophoria is often small, and there may not be a need for treatment unless an exotropia develops.

2.19 Intermittent exotropia

This is the most common type of exodeviation and can be latent or intermittent and usually present before the age of 5 years. The deviation is associated with fatigue, stress, and periods of relative inattention. Initially, the deviation tends to be greater for distance (intermittent distant exotropia—IDEX) than near, and later, the extent is similar irrespective of relative object's position. The disparity could be due to high AC/A ratio or tenacious proximal fusion which arises from slow relaxation of the fusional mechanism, thus limiting conversion of exophoria to exotropia. Progression to constant exotropia is common though there is usually no associated amblyopia. Management involves assessment using the Newcastle control score [34]. Good control is defined when exotropia manifests only with cover test with resumption of vision without blink/refixation. Fair control is defined when exotropia manifests after cover test and fusion resumes with blinking or refixation. Poor control is defined as spontaneous manifestation of exotropia and remaining for extended period. The degree of deviation is assessed at a distance using prism and cover test. Patients' with high AC/A will have less deviation with +3.00 diopters. Intermittent esotropia can be classified based on observed differences in prism and alternate cover tests for near and distance. In the basic type, the deviation is the same for distance and near. In divergence excess, the deviation is greater for distance than near, and convergence insufficiency is present when the deviation is greater for near than distance. Nonsurgical management involves providing appropriate refractive correction in patients with myopia, astigmatism, or hyperopia. Minus lenses of 2–4 diopter sphere can be used to stimulate accommodative convergence and delay surgery. Part time patching (4–6 h daily) and alternate day patching can produce some improvement which can be used before surgery. Some clinicians advocate orthoptic treatment consisting of training for diplopia awareness and fusional convergence. Base in can be used as short-term treatment as their long-term use is associated with reduced fusional convergence amplitude. Surgery should be considered when deviation is present more than half of the time and consists of bilateral recession of lateral rectus muscle, or recession of one lateral rectus with ipsilateral medial rectus resection. Bilateral lateral rectus recession could result in postsurgical (consecutive) esotropia usually of less than 15 prism diopters and may require treatment with press-on prism if persistent beyond 4 weeks of postoperative period. Without evidence of slipped muscle, observation over a few months of period is advocated as spontaneous resolution is common. A review has shown that despite the absence of natural history data of IDEX, unilateral surgery appears to be more effective than bilateral surgery [35].

2.20 Other types of exotropia

This includes constant exotropia that could arise from decompensated intermittent or sensory manifest exotropia and can be treated with similar surgical procedure as intermittent exotropia. Infantile exotropia typically present within the first 6 months of life is usually associated with neurological anomalies. Sensory exotropia could arise from disease causing uniocular visual deprivation such as cataract, corneal opacity, gross retinal anomalies, and optic nerve atrophy. Convergence insufficiency esotropia is not common in children.

2.21 Amblyopia

Amblyopia is defined as the reduction of best-corrected visual acuity of one or both eyes that cannot be attributed exclusively to a structural abnormality of the eye. It develops during childhood and results in the interruption of normal cortical visual pathway development and is characterized by a difference in best-corrected visual acuity of two or more lines between the eyes [36]. A study in Asia, Latin America, and Africa indicated a prevalence of 1.52 per 1000 children [37]. In amblyopia, there is reduced visual acuity and contrast sensitivity due to the abnormal processes in the visual cortex [38]. The causes of amblyopia include uncorrected refractive error, strabismus, and obstruction of the visual axis. There is the traditional view that treatment should commence before the age of 8–9 years, and a study suggests that the treatment can extend into early adulthood as the ability of the brain to adjust (plasticity) extends to such period [39]. Treatment involves correction of refractive errors with guidance on consistent use of the prescribed glasses. Children with conditions giving rise to occlusion of the visual axis (cataract, corneal opacity) should have the cause removed without delay. The patients with strabismus should be accessed, and appropriate treatment measures should be instituted. Patching therapy is indicated to encourage the weaker eye take up fixation and realign with the visual cortex. There are various regimes based on hours per day or, alternate days. It is of importance to monitor the child by both clinician and caregiver to assess progress. Penalization can be employed as alternative to patching, and it involves the use of atropine eye drops to blur images in the better eye, thus encouraging the child to use the so-called weaker eye [40].

3. Conclusion

Childhood strabismus strabismus, presenting unit challenges, is evaluation and management. There is poor recollection of medical history and often children are not accompanied to the hospital by their biological parents. Poor knowledge results in misconception and stigmatization of children with squint. Religious and cultural practices coupled with inequity in access to health care could result in amblyopia, thus retarding the child's development.

Acknowledgements

Appreciation to the management of Bayero University Kano—Nigeria for providing an enabling academic environment.

Conflict of interest

None.

Author details

Lawan Abdu
Department of Ophthalmology, Faculty of Clinical Sciences, College of Health Sciences, Bayero University Kano, Nigeria

*Address all correspondence to: lawal1966@yahoo.com

References

[1] American Academy of Ophthalmology. https://www.aao.org/eye-health/diseases/what-is-strabismus

[2] Tsoucalas G, Papaioannou T, Karamanou M. Michael Constantine Psellus (1020-1105 AD) and his definition of strabismus. Strabismus. 2018;**26**(3):155-157

[3] Zampieri F, Marrone D, Zanatta A. Should the annular tendon of the eye be named 'annulus of Zinn' or 'of Valsalva'? Acta Ophthalmologica. 2015;**93**(1):97-99

[4] Sevel D. The origins and insertions of the extraocular muscles: Development, histologic features, and clinical significance. Transactions of the American Ophthalmological Society. 1986;**84**:488-526

[5] Helveston EM. The influence of superior obligue anatomy on function and treatment. The Bielschowsky lecture. Binocular Vision & Strabismus Quarterly. 1999;**14**(1):16-26

[6] https://medicine.academic.ru/160248/Sherrington's_law

[7] American Academy of Ophthalmology. https://aao.org/image/cardinal-position-yoke-muscle

[8] King WM. Binocular coordination of eye movements: Hering's law of equal innervation or uniocular control? The European Journal of Neuroscience. 2011;**33**(11):2139-2146

[9] Sen DK, Malik SRK. Accommodative-convergence over accommodation (AC/A) ratio (in normal Indian subjects). Indian Journal of Ophthalmology. 1972;**20**(4):153-157

[10] https://www.aao.org/bcscsnippetdetail.aspx?id=a52cc91c-02ea-4d90

[11] Tongue AC, Cibis GW. Brückner test. Ophthalmology. 1981;**88**(10):1041-1044

[12] http://eyewiki.aao.org/Cover_Tests

[13] Daniel S. The Maddox rod test: A ten year follow up. American Journal of Ophthalmology. 1963;**55**(3):484-488

[14] Isawumi MA, Ulaikere M, Adejumo OO, et al. Awareness, perceptions and knowledge of strabismus among patients visiting a tertiary eye clinic in Southwest Nigeria. International Ophthalmology. 2014;**34**(5):1037-1042

[15] Bodunde O, Runsewe-Abiodun T, Alabi A, et al. Awareness and perception of strabismus among the youths and women of child-bearing age in a local government in South Western Nigeria: A qualitative study. International Quarterly of Community Health Education. 22 Jul 2016. DOI: 10.1177/0272684X16660025

[16] Azonobi IR, Olatunji FO, Addo J. Prevalence and pattern of strabismus in Ilorin. West African Journal of Medicine. 2009;**28**(4):253-256

[17] Ntim-Amponsah CT, Ofosu-Amaah S. Prevalence of refractive error and other eye diseases in schoolchildren in the Greater Accra region of Ghana. Journal of Pediatric Ophthalmology and Strabismus. 2007;**44**(5):294-297

[18] Mehari ZA, Yimer AW. Prevalence of refractive errors among schoolchildren in rural Central Ethiopia. Clinical and Experimental Optometry. 2013;**96**(1):65-69

[19] Wedner SH1, Ross DA, Balira R, Kaji L, Foster A. Prevalence of eye diseases in primary school children in a rural area of Tanzania. The British Journal of Ophthalmology. 2000;**84**(11):1291-1297

[20] Ebana MC, Bella-Hiag AL, Epesse M. Strabismus in Cameroon. Journal Français D'ophtalmologie. 1996;**19**(11):705-709

[21] Lawan A, Sani M. Clinicopathological pattern and management of retinoblastoma in Kano-Nigeria. Annals of African Medicine. 2011;**10**(3):214-219

[22] Susan C, Rohit V, Kristina T. The joint writing committee for the multi-ethnic pediatric eye disease study and the Baltimore pediatric eye disease study groups. Ophthalmology. Nov;**118**(11):2251-2261

[23] Robert JB, George SE, Sprague EH. At the crossing: Pediatric ophthalmology and strabismus. In: Proceedings of the 52nd Annual Symposium of the New Orleans Academy of Ophthalmology; New Orleans, LA, USA. The Hague, Netherlands: Kugler Publications; 2004. pp. 99-110

[24] Eustis HS, Nussdorf JD. Inferior oblique overaction in infantile esotropia: Fundus extorsion as a predictive sign. Journal of Pediatric Ophthalmology and Strabismus. 1996;**33**(2):85-88

[25] Shirabe H, Mori Y, Dogru M, et al. Early surgery for infantile esotropia. British Journal of Ophthalmology. 2000;**84**:536-538

[26] Robert PR. Update on accommodative esotropia. Optometry. 2008;**79**(8):422-431

[27] Mulvihill A, MacCann A, Flitcroft I, et al. Outcome in refractive accommodative esotropia. The British Journal of Ophthalmology. 2000;**84**(7):746-749

[28] Davis KC, Cynthis WA, Evelyn AP, et al. Early onset refractive accommodative esotropia. JAAPOS. 1992;**2**(5):275-278

[29] Wook KK, Sung YK, Soolienah R, et al. The analysis of AC/A ratio in nonrefractive accommodative esotropia treated with bifocal glasses. Korean Journal of Ophthalmology. 2012;**26**(1):39-44

[30] Mohney BG. Acquired non-accommodative esotropia in childhood. Journal of AAPOS. 2001;**5**(2):85-89

[31] Paul C. Childhood cataract in sub-Saharan Africa. Saudi Journal of Ophthalmology. 2012;**26**(1):3-6

[32] Lawan A. Primary congenital glaucoma in Kano, northern Nigeria. African Journal of Paediatric Surgery. 2007;**4**(2):75-78

[33] Lenart TD, Lambert SR. Slipped and lost extraocular muscles. Ophthalmology Clinics of North America. 2001;**14**(3):433-442

[34] Haggerty H, Richardson S, Hrisos S, et al. The Newcastle Control Score: A new method of grading the severity of intermittent distance exotropia. British Journal of Ophthalmology. 2004;**88**(2):233-235

[35] Sarah RH, Lawrence G. Interventions for intermittent exotropia. Cochrane Database of Systematic Reviews. 2013;**5**:CD003737

[36] https://www.aao.org/disease-review/amblyopia-introduction

[37] Gilbert CE, Ellwein LB. Refractive Error Study in Children Study Group. Prevalence and causes of functional low vision in school-age children: Results from standardized population surveys in Asia, Africa, and Latin America. Investigative Ophthalmology & Visual Science. 2008;**49**(3):877-881

[38] Levi DM. Linking assumptions in amblyopia. Visual Neuroscience. 2013;**30**(5-6):277-287

[39] Levi DM. Visual processing in amblyopia: Human studies. Strabismus. 2006;**14**(1):11-19

[40] Osborne DC, Greenhalgh KM, Evans MJE, et al. Atropine penalization versus occlusion therapies for unilateral amblyopia after the critical period of visual development: A systematic review. Ophthalmology and Therapy. 2018;7(2):323-332

Chapter 6

Congenital Nasolacrimal Duct Obstruction and the Visual System

Adnan Aslam Saleem

Abstract

Congenital nasolacrimal duct obstruction (CNLDO), previously considered a benign disease, affects 20% of the children globally. It is described by a collection of symptoms in which continuous epiphora and intermittent discharge are present in either one or both the eyes. CNLDO usually resolves in most healthy infants in the first few couple of months; however, it may persist for a number of years in some children. There has been a lot of recent deliberation on how a constant watery eye affects the visual development during the phase of emmetropization in children. A connection between CNLDO and anisometropia has been hypothesized. Multiple factors which include developmental and environmental aspects are thought to play a contributory role in the development of anisometropia by and large; particularly hypermetropic anisometropia, raising the chances of developing amblyopia in children with CNLDO. Published literature on CNLDO had shown inconclusive evidence on this anecdotal propinquity. This chapter discusses CNLDO; etiology, pathogenesis, treatment modalities, surgical intervention, and its role in inducing refractive errors; and its propensity to cause amblyopia.

Keywords: congenital nasolacrimal duct obstruction, anisometropia, refractive status, amblyopia

1. Introduction

Tears are words that need to be written (*Paulo Coelho*). Tears physiology and fluid dynamic are intricate and multifaceted. Tears are produced by the main and accessory lacrimal glands and drain medially into the puncta, then flow through the canaliculi to the lacrimal sac, and then through the nasolacrimal duct (NLD) into the nose. Contraction of the orbicularis muscles creates a pumping action that facilitates the flow of tears through the lacrimal system. Congenital nasolacrimal duct obstructions (CNLDO) are one of the most common cases seen in pediatric ophthalmology clinics. CNLDO occurs in 5–15% of full-term newborns [1]. CNLDO is characterized by epiphora and intermittent discharge. CNLDO remains the most common cause of epiphora in infants. It is usually unilateral or asymmetric and is largely due to a persistent membrane at the level of Hasner valve. The valve of Hasner is located at the distal end of the nasolacrimal duct where it enters the inferior meatus lateral to the inferior turbinate.

The valve of Hasner obstruction occurs due to unfinished canalization, a process that begins in the 12th week of gestation and is completed by the 24th week. An incidence of 35–73% has been reported for imperforate NLDs in full-term infants, with a preponderance opening up spontaneously during the first couple of weeks of life [2]. The nasolacrimal duct normally canalizes from proximal to distal, so the distal portion is often last to open up. Therefore, premature infants conceivably have higher rates of CNLDO. However, because tear production does not take place almost near term, these infants mostly do not exhibit the symptoms of epiphora. Infants with CNLDO present with excessive tearing or mucoid discharge from the eyes due to blockage of the nasolacrimal duct system, which can result in maceration of the of the eyelid skin and local infections. On examination, there is an increased tear meniscus and there may be stickiness or crusting on the lashes. Secondary infection is common in CNLDO due to the stasis of lacrimal sac contents, proximity of the sinuses, and a rich lymphatic and vascular system within the submucosa of the lacrimal sac.

2. Initial assessment

It is important to note that typically, CNLDO does not usually cause much discomfort to children. Affected infants are otherwise well and act normally despite the presence of noteworthy overflow of tears and mucopurulent discharge. If infants have photophobia or other signs of chronic irritation, they should be checked carefully for signs of glaucoma, keratopathy, or epiblepharon, i.e., other factors of pediatric epiphora must be ruled out. The absence of corneal and conjunctival abnormalities is an important factor in establishing a diagnosis of CNLDO. Other causes of epiphora such as acute conjunctivitis, congenital anomalies of the upper lacrimal drainage system (punctal or canalicular atresia or agenesis), entropion, and triachiasis also must be evaluated. The most important entity in the differential diagnosis of CNLDO/epiphora would be infantile glaucoma. NLDO may be confused with glaucoma by primary care physicians due to the presence of epiphora. It is important to check intraocular pressure, corneal diameters, and cup to disk ratio to rule out this condition.

It is recommended to do a fluorescein disappearance test (FDT) on all children with epiphora as it provides evidence to support a diagnosis of lacrimal outflow obstruction. Fluorescein 1% is instilled into each lower conjunctival fornix. The child sits on the parent's lap while the cobalt blue light of a slit lamp is used to illuminates the eyes. Cobalt blue light of an ophthalmoscope can be alternatively used. The tear meniscus is evaluated at 2, 5, and 10 minutes. Each eye is graded at 0, 1, 2, or 3 (0 = fluorescein completely gone, 3 = no fluorescein gone). Normally, the fluorescein disappears by 5 minutes but the dye remains in the conjunctival cul-de-sac in children with obstruction. Mild pressure on the lacrimal sac produces regurgitation of fluorescein-stained tears, particularly in those with a mucocele. This test visibly demonstrates the nature of the problem to the parents and provides practical time to discuss the cause and management of CNLDO. The fluorescein dye disappearance test can reliably confirm lacrimal duct obstruction noninvasively, with a sensitivity of 90% and a specificity of 100% [3]. In most centers, FDT has become the preferred tool for diagnosis of CNLDO.

Approximately 90% infants with CNLDO experience spontaneous resolution before the age of 1 year. It becomes symptomatic in merely 5–6% of infants [4]. Probabilities of spontaneous resolution by 12 months of age are 80–90%, at 3 months of age, 68–75%, at 6 months of age, and 36–57% at 9 months of age [5]. Bilateral symptoms are present in 14.0–33.8% of patients with CNLDO, all of which either spontaneously resolve simultaneously or within 3 months of contralateral resolutions. In cases of bilateral CNLDO, when epiphora in one eye settles spontaneously during 10–12 months of ages, it is rational to monitor the child for further 3 months as spontaneous resolution can occur in a substantial percentage of children after 1 year of age [6].

Congenital dacryocystoceles are an uncommon variant of CNLDO, typically seen at birth or shortly after birth as a blue-colored cystic mass over the lacrimal sac. The valve of Hasner again is the most frequent site obstruction due to incomplete canalization. A congenital dacryocystocele accompanies CNLDO in approximately 0.1% of infants. Children with Down syndrome, craniosynostosis, Goldenhar sequence, clefting syndromes, hemifacial microsomia, and midline facial anomalies are at an increased risk for CNLDOs. Although most cases of CNLDO are diagnosed clinically, some conditions especially craniofacial malformations or Down syndrome, the bony obstruction at the CNLDO can be confirmed with computed tomography (CT Scans). Dacryocystocele (where both proximal and distal lacrimal system are obstructed) commonly results in dacryocystitis (or, rarely, neonatal respiratory obstruction) at birth, it necessitates surgical intervention following diagnostic imaging.

3. Initial Management

The treatment of CNLDO is, at first, conservative. Conservative treatment consists of nasolacrimal massage, warm compresses, and topical antibiotics for secondary infections. Massage of the lacrimal sac increases the hydrostatic pressure within the sac thereby breaking open the distal membrane. The most important aspect of conservative treatment is educating the parents, providing reassurance and information about the etiology, and natural history of CNLDO. Printed leaflets that provide information for the parent are very useful. Parents should be encouraged to clean the lids and lashes with cooled boiled water or normal saline and to lightly express the contents of the lacrimal sac. This maintains flow in the system and prevents stagnation, reducing any sticky discharge. Method of the massage should be explained to the parents. Parents find this difficult and need clear instructions. They should press on the sac below the medial canthus with their little finger multiple times per day if possible. Vaseline or liquid paraffin should be applied to the periocular skin to protect and treat any areas of redness or broken skin.

Antibiotic eye drops in CNLDO should only be used when it is accompanied by signs of conjunctivitis. It is somewhat common practice in some centers that topical antibiotics are used in combination with conservative therapy for CNLDO. However, there is no evidence indicative of the fact that antibiotic eye drops appreciably facilitates the resolution of CNLDO. Conjunctival bacterial flora in CNLDO patients is almost identical to those in the normal pediatric population and the use of antibiotic eye drops may cause normal bacterial flora to be substituted with a drug resistant flora. As infants have immune system that is in flux and is not geared-up to remove resistant bacteria they may possibly become carriers of resistant bacteria. Thus, antibiotic eye drops are completely unnecessary in conservative therapy for simple CNLDO [7].

3.1 Surgical management

Intervention is usually done when CNLDO becomes persistent and/or once the child is older than 1 year of age. Probing the nasolacrimal duct to open the membranous obstruction at the distal nasolacrimal duct is the preferred initial management. Probing can be performed without anesthesia in the office setting, but it is usually preferred to do the procedure under general anesthesia (GA) in the operating room. The benefit of GA is less discomfort and the ability to perform additional procedures if other abnormalities are found while the child is under GA. Probing aims to solve the symptoms of epiphora/discharge by clearing up the membranous obstruction; however, it may not be able to relieve the obstruction if it is due to protrusion of the bone of inferior turbinate into the NLD or when the NLD is swollen due to inflammatory processes such as dacryocystitis. Moreover, probable complications with probing are; false passage formation, injury to the NLD, puncta, canaliculi, bleeding, laryngospasm, and rarely aspiration.

While obstruction is mostly located at the valve of Hasner, obstruction may be anywhere along the route. Surgical intervention consists of the introduction of a flexible metal probe into the nasolacrimal duct to open it. A probe is placed into the nasolacrimal duct and passed into the nose. Following probing the nasolacrimal system is irrigated to assess its patency. This is usually done with normal saline tagged with fluorescein dye. If fluorescein dye can be picked-up by suction from the pharynx, probing can be considered successful. Postoperative tobramycin-dexamethasone eye drops are used four times a day for 2–3 weeks. If after 6 weeks, there is no improvement in signs or symptoms, probing and syringing (P&S) can be repeated. Endoscopic inspection with a nasal scope during P&S is recommended; especially if it is being done the second time, to identify anatomical anomalies and to ensure accurate probe configuration. Various studies show a success rate of 90–95% after initial probing [8–11].

The timing of initial probing is debatable and varies between surgeons and centers. Some surgeons recommend early intervention. Their concern is that prolonged epiphora is annoying to both child and parents. More importantly, a delay in treatment may increase the risk of infections and long-term damage to the system resulting in inferior success rates of simple probing. In countries where pediatric ophthalmic care is limited to a few urban centers; where children present late with complex CNLDO and where there is a high probability the child will not show up for a follow-up, an early probing can be justified to some extent.

Typically, it is thought that the older the child at the time of probing, the less successful the probing will be. Studies have reported variable success rates of probing and syringing when done in older children. A success rate of 94% was reported by Havins and Wilkins for probing done in children less than 8 months compared to 56% in children age 18 months and older [12]. Sturrock reported 86% success when probing was done in children less than 1 year compared to 72% between 1 and 2 years of age and 42% for more than 2 years of age [13]. Katowitz and Welsh reported success rates of 76.4% in 13–18 month old children; however, the cure rates fall to 33.3% in children over 2 years [9].

Mannor et al. found a negative association between the age and success rates of P & S. Contrary to this, Robb, Zwaan, and El-Mansoury found more than 90% success rate in late as well as very late probing [10, 14, 15]. Robb found no difference in cure rate with increasing age and noted an overall success rate of 92% varying from 88.9 to 96.8% at different age intervals up to and beyond 3 years of age [16]. Honavar reported a success rate of 75.0% up to 4 years of age, after which it fell to 42.9% in children older than 4 years [17]. Casady reported success rates of 85% for probing in children more than 18 months of age [18].

Factors besides increasing patient age that are associated with decreased success rates for probing are severe symptoms, bilateral symptoms, canalicular stenosis, atonic sac, and non-membranous CNLDO. A recent Cochrane review assessing the effects of probing for CNLDO showed that the effects and cost of immediate versus deferred P & S for CNLDO are uncertain. Patients with unilateral CNLDO may have improved success from immediate P & S in the clinic. Limiting factors in these studies were; sample sizes of participated children in these trials were small and researchers examined outcomes at different points in time. They conclude that deciding whether to perform the procedure and its best possible timing will entail well-run clinical trials [19].

If the preliminary probing and syringing fails, one may perform; as discussed before, a secondary probing or an additional procedure. Second probing can be repeated four to six after the initial procedure. Cure rates of second probing are greatly decreased because unsuccessful first probing can result in cicatricial strictures or a false passage [20]. The two main secondary procedures are balloon dacryoplasty and silicone tube intubation.

During balloon dacryoplasty, a stent with a balloon at its distal end is passed into the distal nares, the balloon is inflated (usually couple of times), then deflated and removed. The aim is to widen the distal duct and decrease obstruction. The primary advantage of balloon dacryoplasty is that no stent material is left in the lacrimal system and therefore stent removal is not required. Balloon dacryoplasty is particularly useful for patients with diffuse stenosis of the distal NLD. Success rates for balloon dacryoplasty as a primary procedure are as high as 94%; however, the procedure is costly; nevertheless it may have its benefit in intractable cases [21, 22]. Furthermore, the role of balloon dacryoplasty in the management of CNLDO needs further evaluation and assessment.

Intubation is necessary in cases with lacrimal canalicular stenosis after probing. The silicone tube prevents the formation of granulation-related obstruction around the newly patent tract. Bicanalicular or monocanalicular silicone intubation of the nasolacrimal duct can be used as a primary or secondary procedure. Intubation should take place under GA after the nose has been prepared with decongestant. It is recommended that a nasal endoscopic guidance system is used to view the inferior meatus [23]. The lacrimal system should be probed first to ensure that the tubes have an anatomical passage. Tubes come with a metal introducer and one end should be placed through the system via the upper canaliculus, into the sac and down the nasolacrimal duct into the inferior meatus from where it should be retrieved under endoscopic view. The other end of the tube is inserted in exactly the same way through the lower canaliculus. The ends are tied securely with multiple square knots inside the nose and trimmed. Postoperative treatment consists of a topical antibiotic and steroid preparation for 2–3 weeks.

Possible complications of intubation include canalicular cheese-wiring, superiorly/inferiorly dislocation, infection, and scarring of any part of the nasolacrimal drainage system. Silicone tube stents if removed too early may result in the recurrence of obstruction. Breakage or prolapse of the tube may cause corneal abrasions [24]. Retrieval of the probe is sometimes difficult during intubation and during instrumental manipulation required during it may damage the nasal mucosa and turbinate [25]. The timing of removing the tube is contentious, but the suggested time is anywhere between 6 weeks and 18 months [26]. Leaving a tube in situ for about 6 months may attain better success rates compared to removing it earlier [27]. A study reports that early removal of tube in children younger than 2 years did not reduce the success rates of intubation [28]. Long-term intubation is associated with a higher occurrence of breakage, dislodgement, migration, dislocation, or prolapse. Tubes in almost all the cases are removed under GA through the nose. The tube is cut at the medial canthus and removed under direct vision to prevent aspiration of the tube. This system is then irrigated to remove any debris and to verify patency.

Its success rate of intubation range from 62 to 100% but in general, they decrease with increasing age [29, 30]. A study reported success rates for intubation stratified by patient age. The success rate for intubation in children aged 12–24 months was 91.3%, which reduced to 85.5% in those aged 24–36 months and to 79.6% in those aged 36–48 months [31]. Several studies have explored the effectiveness of intubation as a main treatment modality in older subgroup of children because of the decrease in success rates for late probing. Although the success rate was high; none of the studies included a control group.

The bicanalicular device has a silicone tube with a flexible metal probe on each end. Each separate end is introduced into the upper or lower punctum and then retrieved from the nose. Bicanalicular stents pass through both the upper and lower canaliculus and typically create a closed circuit. Bicanacular system intubates the upper and lower canaliculi connecting via the common canaliculus or the lacrimal sac thereby intubating the entire nasolacrimal drainage system with the circuit being open or closed in the nose. Examples of Bicanacular stent include Crawford stent, Ritleng stent, Pigtail/Donut stent, and Kaneka Lacriflow stent.

Monocanalicular stents do not provide a closed loop system, but only intubates either the upper or lower canaliculus. Examples of monocanalicular stents include Monoka Stent and Jones Tube. Both monocanalicular and bicanalicular intubations are effective methods for treating CNLDO. Monocanalicular intubation has the advantage of a lower incidence of canalicular slit formation, technical ease of insertion, and easier tube removal. Moreover, the tubing does not threaten the unprobed part of the lacrimal drainage system [32]. Bicanalicular intubations may be a better treatment for the patients with incomplete complex CNLDO [33].

A met-analysis in 2016 showed that the results of immediate and deferred P & S did not vary in their success rates. There was no difference in between the success rates of balloon dilation and intubation. Monocanalicular and bicanalicular intubation had similar success and dislocation rates. Therefore, the preference of a particular procedure on the treatment of CNLDO should be discussed in detail with parents by the concerned surgeon to achieve the best possible results [34].

In cases where all above measures fail or in complex CNLDO, some surgeons perform additional procedures such as turbinate fracture or dacryocystorhinostomy (DCR). DCR is done provided the obstruction is distal to the lacrimal sac. DCR represents a last resort for patients in whom; multiple procedures have failed, complex CNLDO, or in whom there is obstruction secondary to bony obstruction, dacryocystitis, dacryocystocele, older children, or craniofacial dysmorphism. Infracture of the inferior turbinate, usually done with a periosteal elevator or a hemostat, is used to decrease the resistance of drainage in the distal nasolacrimal duct. It is mostly useful for patients who have an exceedingly tight space between the inferior turbinate and nasal wall. It also allows for better visualization of the inferior meatus during endoscopic surgery. The success rate of inferior turbinate fracture alone is 83% [35]. Although a combination of probing with intubation results in good cure rates of 88–100%, the success rate for a combined inferior turbinate fracture and probing is no different to that for simple probing [36].

Conventional/external DCR is carried out through skin incision, the lacrimal sacs are exposed, an osteotomy is made through the nasal bone, flaps are created between the lacrimal sac and the nasal mucosa and then tube is placed which serves as a stent. Laser DCR is a substitute; the ostium is created by means of a laser which is placed through the canaliculus just adjacent to the nasal bone. An endoscope is mostly used during laser DCR. Nasolacrimal stents are placed at the end of the procedure. External and endoscopic DCR have excellent success rates, comparable to those of adult DCRs [37]. Endoscopic DCR can avoid a cutaneous scar and disruption of the medial canthal anatomy, but a pediatric endoscopic DCR is technically more demanding because of the poor visualization afforded by small nostrils and closer proximity of the operative field to the base of the skull [38].

Pediatric DCR has high success rates of 88–96% for external DCR and 82–92% for endoscopic DCR [39]. Rapidly altering anatomy, ill-defined anatomical landmarks, and aggravated growth of scar tissue have been suggested as possible factors that could influence surgical outcomes in pediatric DCR. On top, because of a narrowed nasal cavity there is a propensity toward development of postoperative adhesions between the rhinostomy site and the nasal septum; the use of a silicone tubes in pediatric DCR may avert this obstruction and consequently ensure better surgical outcomes [40].

4. CNLDO and its effect on the visual system

CNLDO has long been considered as a benign condition that does not influence visual development. CNLDO has been at the hub of current debate on its proposed relationship with anisometropia, strabismus, and amblyopia. The persistent tearing caused by CNLDO distorts retinal images by producing a blur, thus defocusing the retinal image thereby adversely influencing the process of physiological emmetropization. This interference with the physiological emmetropization has possibly led to frequent findings of anisometropia in various studies.

The role of focused retinal images in the physiological emmetropization has been discussed by Wright [41]. Newborns are hyperopic having a short axial length relative to the refractive power of the cornea and lens. During the first few months of life rapid growth in axial length (AL) occurs with subsequently decreases the hypermetropia. The retinal image comes in clear focus through "emmetropization." Various studies have shown that growth of the eye after birth and the development of its refractive capabilities are dependent on vision-dependent retinal mechanisms. A basic observation is that a continuous image blur on the retinal cells in a new born can result in lengthening of the axial length thus inducing myopia. The axiom is that when we are born the AL of the eye is short; therefore, the eye is hypermetropic and image blur on the retinal tissue in early life kindles AL elongation until image clarity is achieved by proper focusing of light rays. Raviola and Wiesel concluded that when visual input is deprived, as seen in cases where there is a dense corneal opacity or ptotic/closed eyelids, the eye has a tendency toward myopia [42]. Even if the eyelids are completely closed, more than 20% of light is still passed on to the retina [43]. The influence of a blur images is so immense that (in a study done on chicks) if only half the retinal image is blurred, then only that half of the globe will lengthen [44].

In comparison to blurred images, if there is no stimulation of light, studies show that it slows down the progress of blurred induced myopia and AL elongation. In theory, clearing up the image blur would abolish the stimulus of image blur on AL elongation, thereby retarding AL growth and the process of emmetropization, thereby causing hypermetropia [45]. In addition to the influence of AL elongation by blurred image stimulation of the retina, it seems that intrinsic growth of the eye is disengaged from visual input. AL elongation and thickness of the choroid alterations occur in diurnal pattern. In general, AL elongates and choroid thickens during the day and dawdle downs at night signifying a circadian rhythm. This suggests that the eye has an intrinsic growth rate that will occur in the absence of visual input [46].

No cause-effect relationship linking CNLDO and anisometropia has been studied and the precise method by which CNLDO might cause refractive error, anisometropia, and amblyopia is indistinct. As discussed, the proper focusing of images on the retina early in life is vital for emmetropization. It is indefinite what part, if any; persistent tearing has on visual development, refractive status, and amblyopia. Several authors have recently described an association between CNLDO and the development of amblyopia and strabismus secondary to anisometropia [47–49]. The major visual concern in CNLDO is the presence of significant anisometropia during vital period of visual development in these infants.

CNLDO rarely, if ever, results in complete visual obstruction. Besides, early unilateral visual deprivation as discussed before has been linked with myopia not hypermetropia [42, 50]. It is postulated that accumulation of discharge, excessive tears, and antibiotic ointments may result in deformation of retinal images. This image disparity may lead to a lack of appropriate emmetropization process and as a result the repeated finding of anisometropia in the affected eye. It is also proposed that this anisometropia is refractory. However, recent studies reveal that this is not necessarily true [51], which will be discussed in a while.

4.1 Visual system, anisometropia, and amblyopia

An estimated 285 million people around the world are visually impaired; 19 million are children below the age of 14 years. Childhood visual impairment is estimated to be the second leading cause of the burden due to blindness [52]. Forty percent of childhood blindness is preventable; 12 million children are visually impaired merely because of refractive errors. Uncorrected refractive errors lead to amblyopia and strabismus [53, 54]. Anisometropia is one of the major causes of amblyopia. Visual disabilities in children are also more intricate compared to adults thus preventing visual impairment in children in resource-poor countries is one of the key components of VISION 2020 the Right to Sight.

The significance of anisometropia as a source of amblyopia is well documented. Amblyopia risk factors based on *American Association for Pediatric Ophthalmology and Strabismus* (AAPOS) criteria include: anisometropia (spherical or cylindrical) >1.5 diopters; any manifest strabismus; hypermetropia >3.5 diopters in any meridian: myopia magnitude >3.0 diopters in any meridian: any media opacity >1 mm; astigmatism >1.5 diopters at 90 or 180° >1.0 diopters in oblique axis (more than 10° from 90 or 180°) and ptosis ≤1 mm margin reflex distance (MRD) [55]. Although binocular single vision (BSV) develops at the age of 2 years, the fixation reflex is not fully established until the age of 9 years. Visual acuity remains in a state of flux prior to this age predisposing the child to anisometropia, strabismus, and amblyopia. In a population-based study on 961 children with amblyopia, the author found the cause to be strabismus in 57%, anisometropia in 17%, and combination of two in 27% patients [56].

Donahue suggests that 1D of anisometropia can be considered as clinically significant anisometropia [57]. Nevertheless due to individual physiologic variability's, amblyopia can even be seen with milder degree of anisometropia. The prevalence of anisometropia in the general pediatric population ranges from 2.3 to 3.4%, based on literature review [58]. Amblyopia has been reported to occur in approximately 1.6–3.6% of the normal population [51, 58]. The prevalence is even higher in medically underserved populations with reported rate as high as 22.7% [59]. The population-based Multi-ethnic Pediatric Eye Disease Study found that 78% of African American and Hispanic children had amblyopia which was traced back to be due to anisometropia [60]. A population-based Baltimore Pediatric Eye Disease Study was conducted on the White and African-American Children. This study concluded that 32% of cases of amblyopia were attributed to anisometropia [61].

Studies on the prevalence of anisometropia (greater and equal to 1D between two eyes) reveal that 2.3–3.4% of pediatric population aged 5–11 years is affected [62, 63]. Drover et al. showed the prevalence of anisometropia to be at 1.4% in the studied pediatric population (mean age 4.2 years) [64]. Huynh et al. study conducted in Sydney, concluded an anisometropic prevalence of 1.6–2.4% (mean age 6.7 years) [65]. Shih and colleagues conducted a population survey in Taiwan and found an anisometropic prevalence ranging from 7.2 to 9.3% in older children (age, 7–18 years) [66]. Studies show that anisometropia is an identifiable amblyogenic factor in 37% of cases and present concurrently with strabismus in an additional 24% of clinical populations [67].

Apart from refractive errors, a variety of risk factors increase the likelihood of amblyopia. A study showed that 28.7% of children whose parents had known strabismus were also found to have strabismus, a known amblyopia risk factor; this suggests a hereditary risk factor [68]. Low birth weight (<2499 g) and severe mental handicap are established risk for developing amblyopia [69]. Further risk factors include capillary hemangiomas of the eyelids, ptosis, blepharophimosis, craniosynostosis, and hydrocephalus. Socioeconomic factors also increase the risk of developing amblyopia. Children from underprivileged background, such as homeless kids and those coming from homes where either parents smoke, have a high prevalence of amblyopia [70, 71].

Amblyopia is clinically significant because it is one of the main causes of visual loss in children. Amblyopia is also of central interest because it suggestive of diminished neuronal activity that occurs when normal visual growth is interrupted. Amblyopia affords an idyllic template for understanding when and how a plastic brain may be used for functional recovery. Impaired stereoscopic depth perception is the most common deficit associated with amblyopia under ordinary binocular viewing conditions. This impairment may have a substantial impact on visuomotor tasks and difficulties in playing sports in children. Furthermore, impaired stereopsis may also limit career options for amblyopes. Stereopsis is more affected in strabismic than in anisometropic amblyopia. Recovery of stereoacuity may require more vigorous treatment protocols in strabismic than in anisometropic amblyopia. Individuals with strabismic amblyopia have a very low probability of improvement with monocular training; however, they get on well with dichoptic training (promising new therapeutic approach to amblyopia, which employs simultaneous and separate stimulation of both eyes) than with monocular training and much better with direct stereo-training [72, 73].

Thus, Anisometropia primarily disturbs binocularity thereby causing reduced stereoacuity. Development of stereoacuity is interrelated to similarity in the refractive status of the fellow eyes; fine motor skills which require swiftness and precision of movements are defective in amblyopic children. Therefore, management of anisometropic amblyopia is more prolonged and complex, especially if it is accompanied with strabismus [74]. In distinction to strabismic and deprivational amblyopia, anisometropic amblyopia is more frequently asymptomatic and detected at an older age; only 15% of affected children are diagnosed before they are 5 years of age [75].

Studies demonstrate that the most important factors in treatment results are age and depth of amblyopia that are directly related to the degree of anisometropia [76]. Therefore, as the child gets older, management becomes more complex and time consuming particularly in hypermetropic anisometropes in whom a less encouraging treatment results are seen, in contrast to myopes. It is suggested that in anisometropic subjects, amblyopia is less severe in children younger than 3 years of age and improvement in visual and stereoacuity is more probable if treatment is initiated prior to this age [77, 78]. Based on repeated finding of anisometropia in CNLDO particularly in unilateral anisometropia it is vital to check refractive status of children with CNLDO to assess visually significant anisometropia at an early age to prevent these children from amblyopia and visual morbidity.

4.2 CNLDO, anisometropia, and amblyogenic potential

First Chalmers and later Ellis questioned the relationship between CNLDO and visual maturation. Chalmers found anisometropia in 3.8%, in eyes with CNLDO; all their subjects were hypermetropic in the affected eye [79]. Ellis found no appreciable increased incidence of amblyopia (1.6%) in a large series of 2249 patients with NLDO compared with controls. They also found no correlation between refractive error and NLDO, including no significant increase in the incidence of anisometropia [80].

In our study, the prevalence of anisometropia (greater than 1.5 D) in NLDO patients of 13.7% is approximately thrice that of the general population [81]. It is also higher than reported studies on this subject matter [47, 48, 79–81]. Similarly, a study of around 1200 CNLDO patients found twice the rate of anisometropia in the unilateral CNLDO patients (7.6%) compared with bilateral NLDO patients (3.6%) that the rate of anisometropia and amblyopia is greater in NLDO patients. Anisometropia occurred at a greater rate in unilateral NLDO patients compared with bilateral NLDO patients and occurred at a greater rate in this CNLDO cohort than expected in the general pediatric population. Several patients with anisometropia went on to develop clinical amblyopia [47].

Matta et al. reviewed 375 patients with CNLDO and reported that 22% of the children with CNLDO had amblyopia risk factors [48]. Piotrowski and colleagues described a high prevalence (9.8%) of anisometropia with or without amblyopia in an 8-year consecutive case series which included 305 children with CNLDO [49]. Furthermore, Eshraghi and colleagues studied 433 cases with CNLDO that underwent probing. They reported that 5.5% had anisometropia and 9.46% had amblyopia risk factors. They also found more anisometropia in failed probing cases and theorized that structural abnormality may have a part to play in the development of anisometropia [82].

Bagheri et al. evaluated refractive state in children with unilateral CNLDO; they reported that in children aged 4 years and older, the interocular difference between spherical error and spherical equivalent was considerable as compared to children younger than 4 years [83]. Contrary to this, in our study, we found no significant association between the age (in months) of the patients and the interocular difference in sphere, cylinder, and SE of affected and non-affected eyes. However, when we observed the refractive status of children with CNLDO, we found that as the children age increased the prevalence and severity of refractive error and anisometropia increased. We also observed that difference between the affected and fellow eyes was significant in terms of spherical refractive error and spherical equivalent and that hypermetropia was more common in the eye with CNLDO. These findings illustrate that when unilateral CNLDO becomes chronic, the likelihood and severity of hypermetropia increases which as detailed, is a risk factor for amblyopia [81, 84]. This finding is clinically significant, as management and prognosis of amblyopia becomes intricate in older children.

The published literature proposes that the prevalence of anisometropia increases as the nature of the CNLDO becomes more chronic. Our study on bilateral CNLDO shows that the interocular difference in the mean spherical equivalent of children with unilateral CNLDO increases with the age of the patients. This was not the case in the patients with bilateral CNLDO. Therefore, children with chronic obstruction are more prone to be amblyogenic [85]. Hence, timely resolution of the problem is recommended to avoid visual morbidity, i.e., anisometropia and amblyogenicity.

If the anticipated association between CNLDO and anisometropia is refractory and the persistent epiphora, discharge, and topical medication in the conjunctival cul-de-sac is being held responsible in hampering the physiological emmetropization, then early resolution of CNLDO should retard the development of anisometropia and thus save the child from developing anisometropic amblyopia. However, a study found results contrary to this. Recently, Pyi Son studied 244 cases and found that early and spontaneous resolution of CNLDO is more likely to have a higher (not lower) rate of anisometropia compared to spontaneous or surgical resolution [86]. They proposed that the eye with CNLDO proceeds to emmetropization differently than the unaffected eye. Early resolution can hinder the process of emmetropization in the affected eye, making it lag behind the normal eye in achieving emmetropization. These findings negate the fact that anisometropia in CNLDO is transient and refractory. Further studies need to be done to determine the timing of resolution of CNLDO and its effect on the development, progression, and resolution of anisometropia and if present amblyopia. In most studies, including the one we conducted, they did not determine whether anisometropia persisted or not after surgical intervention or in later life. Simon reported that even after CNLDO has improved, anisometropic hypermetropia is a regular finding in patients with a history of unilateral CNLDO [87]. Nevertheless, results of all these studies consistently report high rates of anisometropia which concomitantly has amblyogenic effect.

Even though studies suggest that correction of the refractive error in anisometropia alone results in enhances quality of vision in anisometropic amblyopia, it is usually contemplated that most of cases will need added treatment because refractive error adjustment alone will not be adequate to completely manage the depth of amblyopia. Therefore, patching or pharmacological treatment is often prescribed at the same time or soon after the refractive spectacle correction is given. Concrete evidence, generally from the Pediatric Eye Disease Investigator Group, has established both number of hours per day of patching (according to age) and days per week of atropine use as good penalization technique to improve vision and stereoacuity in amblyopia [88]. The use of glasses alone has also been recognized as an excellent first-line treatment for both anisometropic and strabismic amblyopia. IPad-based dichoptic training has shown promising data for vision rehabilitation in amblyopes. Use of pharmaceutical augmentation of traditional therapies has also been investigated. Several different drugs with unique mechanisms of action are thought to improve the receptiveness to amblyopia therapy. However, no data on new treatment options from evidence-based research has surfaced which proves as being better to conventional therapies in regular clinical practice. Continued research into the use of new technology and comprehending the neuronal basis of amblyopia promises alternate or perhaps improved cures in the near future [89].

Studies mention that emmetropia is achievable in anisometropes with appropriate management [90]. However, the precise cause why studies find high prevalence of anisometropia in subjects even after CNLDO has resolved is still contentious. Nevertheless, the results endorse the fact that patients of CNLDO should be regularly reviewed for refractory status. Furthermore, as shown in our results, in older subjects, the interocular difference becomes more significant compared to younger children; this places them at high risk for developing amblyopia. They are also inclined to poor prognosis in terms of visual recovery. These facts support the benefit of early intervention in CNLDO. However, further studies with larger sample size longer follow-up time is required to establish this effect.

5. Conclusion

CNLDO should be observed and treated conservatively till the child is 1 year old. If CNLDO does not respond to conservative treatment, then they should be promptly treated with probing and syringing. In cases remission two cycles of syringing and probing, intubation is a reasonable treatment option. Surgical procedures should be reserved for complicated cases. Unilateral CNLDO is a risk factor for anisometropia particularly hypermetropic anisometropia with amblyogenic potential. Keeping in view that CNLDO is a common presentation in pediatric ophthalmology clinics, we recommend that all children with CNLDO should be regularly followed, even after the obstruction has anatomically and functionally resolved. These children should undergo cycloplegic refraction on each visit and should be monitored for the development of amblyopia and other ocular abnormalities.

Author details

Adnan Aslam Saleem
Amanat Eye Hospital, Islamabad, Pakistan

*Address all correspondence to: doctoradnansaleem@gmail.com

References

[1] Macewen CJ. Congenital nasolacrimal duct obstruction. Comprehensive Ophthalmol Update. 2006;7:79-87

[2] Shekunov J, Griepentrog GJ, Diehl NN, Mohney BG. Prevalence and clinical characteristics of congenital dacryocystocele. Journal of AAPOS. 2010;**14**:417-420

[3] MacEwen CJ, Young JD. The fluorescein disappearance test (FDT): An evaluation of its use in infants. Journal of Pediatric Ophthalmology and Strabismus. 1991;**28**:302-305

[4] Schnall BM. Pediatric nasolacrimal duct obstruction. Current Opinion in Ophthalmology. 2013;**24**:421-424

[5] Kakizaki H, Takahashi T, Kinoshita S, Shiraki K, Iwaki M. The rate of symptomatic improvement of congenital nasolacrimal duct obstruction in Japanese infants treated with conservative management during the first year of age. Clinical Ophthalmology. 2008;**2**:291-294

[6] Schellini SA, Capanema S, Ribeiro F, Jaqueta E, Padovani CR, Padovani CRP. Spontaneous resolution in congenital nasolacrimal obstruction after 12 months. Seminars in Ophthalmology. 2007;**22**:71-74

[7] Olver J. Paediatric lacrimal surgery. In: Colour Atlas of Lacrimal Surgery. Butterworth-Heinemann: Oxford; 2002. pp. 69-89

[8] Baker JD. Treatment of congenital nasolacrimal duct obstruction. Journal of Pediatric Ophthalmology and Strabismus. 1985;**22**:34-36

[9] Katowitz JA, Welsh MG. Timing of initial probing and irrigation in congenital nasolacrimal duct obstruction. Ophthalmology. 1987;**94**:698-705

[10] Mannor GE, Rose GE, Frimpong-Ansah K, Ezra E. Factors affecting the success of nasolacrimal duct probing for congenital nasolacrimal duct obstruction. American Journal of Ophthalmology. 1999;**127**:616-617

[11] Robb RM. Probing and irrigation for congenital nasolacrimal duct obstruction. Archives of Ophthalmology. 1986;**104**:378-379

[12] Havins HE, Wilkins RB. A useful alternative to silicone intubation in congenital nasolacrimal duct obstruction. Ophthalmic Surgery. 1983;**78**:892-894

[13] Sturrock SM, MacEwen CJ, Young JD. Long-term results after probing for congenital nasolacrimal duct obstruction. The British Journal of Ophthalmology. 1994;**78**:892-894

[14] El-Mansoury J, Calhoun JH, Nelson LB, Harley RD. Results of late probing for congenital nasolacrimal duct obstruction. Ophthalmology. 1986;**93**:1052-1054

[15] Robb RM. Success rate of nasolacrimal duct probing at time intervals after 1 year of age. Ophthalmology. 1998;**105**:1308-1310

[16] Zwaan J. Treatment of congenital nasolacrimal duct obstruction before and after the age of 1 year. Ophthalmic Surgery and Lasers. 1997;**28**:932-936

[17] Honavar SG, Prakash VE, Rao GN. Outcome of probing for congenital nasolacrimal duct obstruction in older children. American Journal of Ophthalmology. 2000;**130**:42-48

[18] Casady DR, Meyer DR, Simon JW, Stasior GO, Zobal-Ratnar JL. Stepwise treatment paradigm for congenital

nasolacrimal duct obstruction. Ophthalmic Plastic and Reconstructive Surgery. 2006;**22**:243-247

[19] Petris C, Liu D. Probing for congenital nasolacrimal duct obstruction. The Cochrane Database of Systematic Reviews. 2017;**7**:CD011109

[20] Young JD, MacEwen CJ, Ogston SA. Congenital nasolacrimal duct obstruction in the second year of life: A multicentre trial of management. Eye. 1996;**10**:485-491

[21] Yusksel D, Ceylan K, Erden O, Kilic¸ S, Duman S. Balloon dilatation for treatment of congenital nasolacrimal duct obstruction. European Journal of Ophthalmology. 2005;**15**:179-185

[22] Goldstein SM, Goldstein JB, Katowitz JA. Comparison of monocanalicular stenting and balloon dacryoplasty in secondary treatment of congenital nasolacrimal duct obstruction after failed primary probing. Ophthalmic Plastic and Reconstructive Surgery. 2004;**20**:352-357

[23] Singh S, Mittal V, Vashist U, Mittal R, Narang P. Utility of intraocular endoscope for lacrimal canaliculi and sac examination. International Ophthalmology. 2018 [Epub ahead of print]

[24] Kapadia MK, Freitag SK, Woog JJ. Evaluation and management of congenital nasolacrimal duct obstruction. Otolaryngologic Clinics of North America. 2006;**39**:959-977

[25] Repka MX. Timing of simple probing for congenital nasolacrimal duct obstruction: Not so simple. JAMA Ophthalmology. 2018 [Epub ahead of print]

[26] Ratliff CD, Meyer DR. Silicone intubation without intranasal fixation for treatment of congenital nasolacrimal duct obstruction. American Journal of Ophthalmology. 1994;**118**:781-785

[27] Leone CR, Van Gemert JV. The success rate of silicone intubation in congenital lacrimal obstruction. Ophthalmic Surgery. 1990;**21**:90-92

[28] Peterson NJ, Weaver RG, Yeatts RP. Effect of short-duration silicone intubation in congenital nasolacrimal duct obstruction. Ophthalmic Plastic and Reconstructive Surgery. 2008;**24**:167-171

[29] Marr JE, Drake-Lee A, Willshaw HE. Management of childhood epiphora. The British Journal of Ophthalmology. 2005;**89**:1123-1126

[30] Mauffray RO, Hassan AS, Elner VM. Double silicone intubation as treatment for persistent congenital nasolacrimal duct obstruction. Ophthalmic Plastic and Reconstructive Surgery. 2004;**20**:44-49

[31] Pediatric Eye Disease Investigator Group. Primary treatment of nasolacrimal duct obstruction with nasolacrimal duct intubation in children younger than 4 years of age. Journal of AAPOS. 2008;**12**:451-455

[32] Komínek P, Cervenka S, Pniak T, Zeleník K, Tomášková H, Matoušek P. Monocanalicular versus bicanalicular intubation in the treatment of congenital nasolacrimal duct obstruction. Graefe's Archive for Clinical and Experimental Ophthalmology. 2011;**249**:1729-1733

[33] Eshraghi B, Jamshidian-Tehrani M, Mirmohammadsadeghi A. Comparison of the success rate between monocanalicular and bicanalicular intubations in incomplete complex congenital nasolacrimal duct obstruction. Orbit. 2017;**36**:215-217

[34] Lin AE, Chang YC, Lin MY, Tam KW, Shen YD. Comparison of treatment for congenital nasolacrimal duct

obstruction: A systematic review and meta-analysis. Canadian Journal of Ophthalmology. 2016;**51**:34-40

[35] MacEwen CJ, Young JDH, Barras CW, Ram B, White PS. Value of nasalendoscopy and probing in the diagnosisand management of children with congenital epiphora. The British Journal of Ophthalmology. 2001;**85**:314-318

[36] Attarzadeh A, Sajjadi M, Owji N, Talebnejad MR, Farvardin M, Attarzadeh A. Inferior turbinate fracture and congenital nasolacrimal duct obstruction. European Journal of Ophthalmology. 2006;**14**:520-524

[37] Hakin KN, Sullivan TJ, Sharma A, Welham RA. Paediatric dacryocystorhinostomy. Australian and New Zealand Journal of Ophthalmology. 1994;**22**:231-235

[38] Barnes EA, Abou-Rayyah Y, Rose GE. Paediatric dacryocystorhinostomy for nasolacrimal duct obstruction. Ophthalmology. 2001;**108**:1562-1564

[39] VanderVeen DK, Jones DT, Tan H, Petersen RA. Endoscopic dacryocystorhinostomy in children. Journal of AAPOS;**5**:143-147

[40] Leibovitch I, Selva D, Tsirbas A, Greenrod E, Pater J, Wormald PJ. Paediatric endoscopic endonasal dacryocystorhinostomy in congenital nasolacrimal duct obstruction. Graefe's Archive for Clinical and Experimental Ophthalmology. 2006;**244**:1250-1254

[41] Wright KW. Text of Ophthalmology. Baltimore, MD: Williams & Wilkins; 1997. pp. 371-376

[42] Raviola E, Wiesel TN. An animal model of myopia. The New England Journal of Medicine. 1985;**312**:1609

[43] Slataper FJ. Age norms of refraction and vision. Archives of Ophthalmology. 1950;**43**:466-481

[44] Guyton DL, Green PR, Scholz RT. Dark-rearing interference with emmetropization in the rhesus monkey. Investigative Ophthalmology and Visual Science. 1989;**30**:761-764

[45] Langford JD, Linberg JV, Blaylock WK, Chao GM. Axial myopia in congenital ptosis: An animal model. Ophthalmic Plastic and Reconstructive Surgery. 1998;**14**:261-265

[46] Nickla DL, Wildsoet CF, Troilo D. Endogenous rhythms in axial length and choroidal thickness in chicks: Implications for ocular growth regulation. Investigative Ophthalmology. 2001;**42**:584-588

[47] Kipp MA, Kipp MA Jr, Struthers W. Anisometropia and amblyopia in nasolacrimal duct obstruction. Journal of AAPOS. 2013;**17**:235-238

[48] Matta NS, Silbert DI. High prevalence of amblyopia risk factors in preverbal children with nasolacrimal duct obstruction. Journal of AAPOS. 2011;**15**:350-352

[49] Piotrowski JT, Diehl NN, Mohney BG. Neonatal dacryostenosis as a risk factor for anisometropia. Archives of Ophthalmology. 2010;**128**:1166-1169

[50] Weiss AH. Unilateral high myopia: Optical components, associated factors, and visual outcomes. British Journal of Ophthalmology. 2003;**87**:1025-1031

[51] Ozgur OR, Sayman IB, Oral Y, Akmaz B. Prevalence of amblyopia in children undergoing nasolacrimal duct irrigation and probing. Indian Journal of Ophthalmology. 2013;**61**:698-700

[52] Stevens GA, White RA, Flaxman SR, Price H, Jonas JB, Keeffe J, et al. Global prevalence of vision impairment and blindness: Magnitude and temporal trends, 1990-2010. Ophthalmology. 2013;**120**:2377-2384

[53] Khandekar R. Visual disabilities in children including childhood blindness. Middle East African Journal of Ophthalmology. 2008;**15**:129-134

[54] Naidoo KS, Leasher J, Bourne RR, Flaxman SR, Jonas JB, Keeffe J, et al. Global vision impairment and blindness due to uncorrected refractive error, 1990-2010. Optometry and Vision Science. 2016;**93**:227-234

[55] American Academy of Ophthalmology Pediatric Ophthalmology/Strabismus Panel. Amblyopia. San Francisco, CA: American Academy of Ophthalmology; 2007 (Preferred Practice Pattern Guidelines)

[56] Woodruff G, Hiscox F, Thompson JR, Smith LK. Factors affecting the outcome of children treated for amblyopia. Eye. 1994;**8**:627-631

[57] Donahue SP. Relationship between anisometropia, patient age and the development of amblyopia. American Journal of Ophthalmology. 2006;**142**:132-140

[58] Simons K. Amblyopia characterization, treatment, and prophylaxis. Survey of Ophthalmology. 2005;**50**:123-166

[59] Soori H, Ali JM, Nasrin R. Prevalence and cause of low vision and blindness in Tehran Province, Iran. The Journal of the Pakistan Medical Association. 2011;**61**:544-549

[60] Multi-ethnic Pediatric Eye Disease Study Group. Prevalence of amblyopia and strabismus in African American and Hispanic children ages 6 to 72 months: the Multi-ethnic Pediatric Eye Disease Study. Ophthalmology. 2008;**115**:1229-1236

[61] Friedman DS, Repka MX, Katz J, et al. Prevalence of amblyopia and strabismus in white and African children age 6 through 71 months: The Baltimore Pediatric eye disease study. Ophthalmology. 2009;**116**:2128-2134

[62] Flom MC, Neumaier RW. Prevalence of amblyopia. Public Health Reports. 1966;**81**:329-341

[63] Peters HB, Blum HL, Betman JW, Johnson F, Fellows V Jr. The Orinda vision study. American Journal of Optometry and Archives of American Academy of Optometry. 1959;**36**:455-469

[64] Drover JR, Kean PG, Courage ML, Adams RJ. Prevalence of amblyopia and other vision disorders in young Newfoundland and Labrador children. Canadian Journal of Ophthalmology. 2008;**43**:89-94

[65] Huynh SC, Wang XY, Ip J, et al. Prevalence and associations of anisometropia and aniso-astigmatism in a population based sample of 6 year old children. The British Journal of Ophthalmology. 2006;**90**:597-601

[66] Shih YF, Hsiao CH, Wen SH, Lin LL, Chen CJ, Hung PT. Prevalence of anisometropia in Taiwanese schoolchildren. Journal of the Formosan Medical Association. 2005;**104**:412-417

[67] Pediatric Eye Disease Investigator Group. The clinical profile of moderate amblyopia in children younger than 7 years. Archives of Ophthalmology. 2002;**120**:281-287

[68] Gigantelli JW. The lacrimal drainage system. In: Yanoff M, Duker JS, editors. Ophthalmology. Philadelphia: Mosby; 1999. p. 17.3

[69] Robaei D, Kifley A, Gole GA, Mitchell P. The impact of modest prematurity on visual function at age 6 years: Findings from a population-based study. Archives of Ophthalmology. 2006;**124**:871-877

[70] Tay T, Martin F, Rowe N, Johnson K, Poole M, Tan K, et al. Prevalence and causes of visual impairment in craniosynostotic syndromes. Clinical & Experimental Ophthalmology. 2006;**34**:434-440

[71] Altintas O, Etus V, Etus H, Ceylan S, Caglar S, Caglar Y. Risk of strabismus and amblyopia in children with hydrocephalus. Graefe's Archive for Clinical and Experimental Ophthalmology. 2005;**243**:1213-1217

[72] Levi DM, Knill DC, Bavelier D. Stereopsis and amblyopia: A mini-review. Vision Research. 2015;**114**:17-30

[73] O'Connor AR, Tidbury LP. Stereopsis: Are we assessing it in enough depth? Clinical & Experimental Optometry. 2018;**101**:485-494

[74] Barrett BT, Bradley A, Candy TR. The relationship between anisometropia and amblyopia. Progress in Retinal and Eye Research. 2013;**36**:120-158

[75] Donahue SP. The relationship between anisometropia, patient age, and the development of amblyopia. Transactions of the American Ophthalmological Society. 2005;**103**:313-336

[76] Caputo R, Frosini R, De Libero C, Campa L, Magro EF, Secci J. Factors influencing severity of and recovery from anisometropic amblyopia. Strabismus. 2007;**15**:209-214

[77] Birch EE. Amblyopia and binocular vision. Progress in Retinal and Eye Research. 2013;**33**:67-84

[78] De Zárate BR, Tejedor J. Current concepts in the management of amblyopia. Clinical Ophthalmology. 2007;**1**:403-414

[79] Chalmers RJ, Griffiths PG. Is congenital nasolacrimal duct obstruction a risk factor for the development of amblyopia? British Orthoptic Journal. 1996;**53**:29-30

[80] Ellis JD, MacEwen CJ, Young JDH. Can congenital nasolacrimal duct obstruction interfere with visual development? A cohort case control study. Journal of Pediatric Ophthalmology and Strabismus. 1998;**35**:81-85

[81] Saleem AA, Siddiqui SN, Wakeel U, Asif M. Anisometropia and refractive status in children with unilateral congenital nasolacrimal duct obstruction. Taiwan Journal of Ophthalmology. 2018;**8**:31-35

[82] Eshraghi B, Akbari MR, Fard MA, Shahsanaei A, Assari R, Mirmohammadsadeghi A. The prevalence of amblyogenic factors in children with persistent congenital nasolacrimal duct obstruction. Graefe's Archive for Clinical and Experimental Ophthalmology. 2014;**252**:1847-1852

[83] Bagheri A, Safapoor S, Yazdani S, Yaseri M. Refractive state in children with unilateral congenital nasolacrimal duct obstruction. Journal of Ophthalmic & Vision Research. 2012;**7**:310-315

[84] Siddiqui SN, Hannan A, Mansoor H, Asif M, Wakeel U. Anisometropia and refractive status in children with bilateral congenital nasolacrimal duct obstruction. Journal of the College of Physicians and Surgeons–Pakistan. 2018;**28**:210-213

[85] Siddiqui SN, Mansoor H, Asif M, Wakeel U, Saleem AA. Comparison of Anisometropia and refractive status in children with unilateral and bilateral congenital nasolacrimal duct obstruction. Journal of Pediatric Ophthalmology and Strabismus. 2016;**53**:168-172

[86] Pyi Son MK, Hodge DO, Mohney BG. Timing of congenital dacryostenosis

resolution and the development of anisometropia. The British Journal of Ophthalmology. 2014;**98**:1112-1115

[87] Simon JW, Ngo Y, Ahn E, Khachikian S. Anisometropic amblyopia and nasolacrimal duct obstruction. Journal of Pediatric Ophthalmology and Strabismus. 2009;**46**:182-183

[88] Kraus CL, Culican SM. New advances in amblyopia therapy I: Binocular therapies and pharmacologic augmentation. The British Journal of Ophthalmology. 2018 [Epub ahead of print]

[89] Kraus CL, Culican SM. New advances in amblyopia therapy II: Refractive therapies. The British Journal of Ophthalmology. 2018 [Epub ahead of print]

[90] Atilla H, Kaya E, Erkam N. Emmetropization in anisometropic amblyopia. Strabismus. 2009;**17**:16-19

Chapter 7

Advances in Vitreoretinal Surgery

Baris Komur

Abstract

Vitreoretinal surgery has been radically changed over the past 10 years by the development of new techniques, smaller gauge instrumentation, and improvements in vitrectomy machines. The indications for vitrectomy have expanded dramatically, and inoperable conditions have become amenable to surgical treatment. In addition to improvements in intraocular instruments, various dyes become available and enable better visualization and a more complete removal of vitreous and membranes. In this chapter, we issued latest developments in the surgical field of retina that enable improved surgical outcomes and less complications.

Keywords: vitrectomy, 23 gauge, 25 gauge, 27 gauge, sutureless, retinal detachment, epiretinal membrane, macular hole, silicone oil, c3f8, sf6

1. Introduction

The introduction of pars plana vitreous surgery in the early 1970s, by Dr. Robert Machemer which was a single-port 17 gauge (1.14 mm) system with a cut rate of less than 400 cuts per minute (cpm), is considered as an important step in surgical treatment of vitreoretinal diseases [1]. For the first time, patients with dense vitreous hemorrhage could achieve some visual improvement. Vitreoretinal surgery has changed a lot from that time, firstly by technological improvements in vitrectomy machines. Three-port vitrectomy, better fluidic controls, faster cut rates, better light sources, and smaller gauges are made available to vitreoretinal surgeons [2]. Secondly new techniques and devices like automated fluid-air exchange, endolaser [3], internal tamponades, and dyes make possible to treat different retinal pathologies with less complications. The advent of 23 and 25 gauge vitrectomy made sutureless surgery possible. Improvements in viewing systems and digital image software processing enable good visualization in difficult situations. These advances have enabled vitreoretinal surgeons to more effectively address different serious sight-threatening retinal conditions, including retinal detachments, epiretinal membranes, macular holes, vitreous hemorrhages, phacoemulsification complications, and subluxated intraocular lenses. In this chapter we will discuss latest developments in vitreoretinal surgery that enables improved surgical outcomes and less complications.

2. Improvements in vitrectomy machines

2.1 New probes

The main vitrectomy probe, during the 1990s and 2000s, is made with spring-driven pneumatic cutting mechanism up to 2500 cpm [4]. In these systems,

IntechOpen

pneumatic pulses push the cutter to one direction, and the passive recoil of a spring returns the blade to its original position. The limitation of this design is in higher cutting rates; the speed of the spring recoil is not enough to return the blade. For these cutters, when cutting rates approach 2500 cpm, the blade could not fully return to the initial position that the vitrector port is open, so a higher proportion of a cutting cycle is spent with the port closed. Duty cycle of vitrectomy cutter refers to proportion of one cutting cycle in which the vitrectomy port is open. This is important because active removal of vitreous only occurs only when the port is open. Current-generation vitrectomy systems can achieve at least 5000–7500 cpm, but with a traditional spring-driven pneumatic cutter, vitreous removal efficiency may not necessarily proportionally increase with higher cut rates. There are currently two strategies to improve this limitation. A dual-pneumatic-driven cutting mechanism uses separate air lines to control opening and closing of the cutter. In this system, duty cycle is not dependent on the passive recoil of springs and also can be set individually. The other strategy is using a two-dimensional cutter (TDC) approach in which a double-sided blade cuts in both the forward and reverse directions to achieve an effective cut rate of 16,000 cpm with higher duty cycle [5]. The high duty cycle is achieved because the port is nearly always open as the blade moves back and forth. In dual-pneumatic systems, however, duty cycle can be controlled independent of the cut rate. Studies comparing 7500 cpm dual-pneumatic and 16,000 cpm TDC cutters against their traditional counterparts (5000 cpm spring-driven probes) have demonstrated the new technology to significantly decrease the core vitrectomy time with TDC cutters reducing surgery time by 34–50% [6, 7]. Recently, a new mechanism using ultrasound to liquefy vitreous has been developed. The ultrasound harmonic vitrector liquefies the vitreous before being aspirated and has been shown to be safe on cadaveric eyes. These vitrectomy probes have the potential advantage of creating almost no traction during vitrectomy [8, 9].

2.2 Endoillumination and chandelier systems

Endoillumination utilizes an optic fiber inserted into the vitreous cavity through one of the vitrectomy ports. The first generation of endoilluminators utilized halogen, mercury vapor, and metal halide light bulb [10]. However, halogen illuminators required more power as 50% of the luminance was lost [11]. Present vitrectomy platforms utilize xenon or light-emitting diode (LED) light sources. Both have significant luminance through small-gauge light probes and considerably longer bulb life. With increased illumination and spectral distribution, concerns about possible retinal phototoxicity with xenon light sources from wavelengths below 450 nm have been raised. For this reason, most manufacturers have incorporated low-wavelength filters to block the blue and ultraviolet light most toxic to the retina [11]. LED light sources appear to be less phototoxic in animal models at the same intensity [12].

Chandelier lighting system is a stationary, wide-angle endoillumination developed for retinal surgery. It allows the surgeon to use the second hand for bimanual surgical manipulations. Chandelier lighting systems can be placed as single or double fibers and are available in 23, 25, 27, and even 29 gauge sizes. Apart from being used in complicated tractional retinal detachments, chandeliers have been used for primary scleral buckles for better identification of retinal breaks with wide-angle viewing systems [13]. Chandelier-guided scleral buckling is an effective alternative technique to the traditional scleral buckling. Another use of chandelier illumination system is utilizing retroillumination to enhance the poor red reflex that is typical in cases of combined cataract surgery and vitrectomy for vitreous hemorrhage [14]. Details of chandelier lighting system uses in surgery are discussed in "Surgical techniques" of this chapter.

3. Smaller gauges and cannulas

3.1 Smaller incision sizes

In the past two decades, following similar trends of smaller instrumentation in phacoemulsification surgery in the anterior segment, the evolution of vitrectomy surgical techniques that had an exciting advance with vitrectomy scleral incision size has gradually decreased from 20 gauge to 23 gauge and eventually to 25 gauge and 27 gauge through transconjunctival incisions [15].

The smaller gauges have some disadvantages at first. Instrumentation was originally so impractical that many experienced surgeons encounter a learning curve transition from 20 gauge to smaller gauge. Like every new innovation, restrictions in instrumentation and refinement of surgical techniques are needed. Some early difficulties were instruments were too flexible, small-gauge endoillumінations were weak, and speed of vitreous removal was slow. Improvements in trocar insertion techniques, vitrectomy machine fluidics, stiffer surgical instruments, and valved cannula systems have largely eliminated these issues. Wide range of different stiffer vitreoretinal microsurgical instruments has now been designed for 23 gauge and 25 gauge vitrectomy systems. These include vitreous cutters, trocars, illumination probes, intraocular forceps, micro vitreoretinal blades, tissue manipulators, aspirating picks, aspirators, soft-tip cannulas, curved scissors, extendable curved picks, extendable curved intraocular laser probes, and diathermy probes [16, 17].

Recent introduction of the 25 gauge and 27 gauge vitrectomy systems has some benefits in terms of surgical technique. The cutting port of these probes is closer to the distal end of the tip which gives access to tighter tissue planes during an epiretinal membrane dissection like in diabetic tractional membranes. This manipulation is better than bimanual approach because no instrument change is needed. Combined with the improvements in surgical techniques and better visualization with wide-angle systems, the vitrectomy probe may be used as forceps, scissor, and delamination spatula when necessary without exit from the eye. When a bimanual approach is necessary, chandeliers usually provide an optimal amount of light even the smaller gauges. In these situations, forceps can delaminate any membrane without the need of scissors.

At present, the smallest sclera incision available is 27 gauge. One factor that may lead to a learning curve for 27 gauge is the relative lack of rigidity in the instruments compared to 25 gauge, particularly the intraocular microforceps. Although the main goal of 27 gauge vitrectomy is to create less traumatic wounds, intraoperative surgical times and complications will likely be reduced with this new technology.

3.2 Valved cannulas

Valved cannula systems permit closed system fluidics by limiting exit of fluid which brings various advantages. Maybe the most critical advantage is the exact intraocular pressure (IOP) control that can be kept up consistently during manipulations in trocars, particularly with new IOP stabilization capabilities of current vitrectomy machines.

With reduced flow and turbulence, valved cannulas offer a potential for decreased vitreous incarceration and fewer intraoperative iatrogenic retinal tears, which has been shown in postmortem rabbit eyes [18].

Valved cannulas have few disadvantages also. First it is more difficult to insert soft-tip instruments trough the trocar. Instruments with shorter and more rigid soft extensions and retractable soft tips are useful for insertion. Secondly extra care must be practiced while injecting extra fluid into system with valved trocars. In particular, injection of perfluorocarbon (PFC) liquid, silicone oil, or gas may require one of the trocars to be open, either by a backflush or another instrument to open the valve, by putting a "chimney" vent or by expelling the valve. A dual-bore injection cannula might be useful to permit departure of liquid trough the other bore during injection. In addition, perfusion at the optic nerve must be persistently observed to prevent excessive IOP rise, during every stage of the surgery.

4. Wide-angle viewing systems

Wide-angle viewing systems (WAVs) are useful fundus observation devices for vitreous surgery, which have been continually developed from the late 1980s based on the indirect ophthalmoscopic principles [19, 20].

Visualization during vitreoretinal surgery is the most important part of the surgery particularly while working on complicated cases. Current WAVs comprise of an indirect ophthalmoscopic lens system for panoramic fundus view. In contact type of WAV, the lens is put on the cornea as a contact lens. In noncontact type of WAV, the lens is placed above the cornea. There is also a prismatic reinverter in the system, which is mounted on microscope or the lens system itself for inverting the fundus view. Contact type of WAVs has a predetermined field angle of view which is dependent on the magnification power of the lens, while noncontact type of WAV angle of view can be adjusted by changing the distance between the lens and cornea. The surgeon can increase magnification of fundus view with two types of WAVs by using zooming function of microscope. The image quality is hypothetically prevalent with the contact type of WAV because of the fact that the aberration and reflection from the cornea can be compensated by putting the contact lens directly on the corneal surface without an interphase [21]. Then again, contact type of WAV frequently needs an accomplished assistant to hold the lens during the surgery.

The WAVs enhance the safety and proficiency of the vitreoretinal surgeries by providing a panoramic view of the retina [21]. Vitreoretinal surgeon can undoubtedly assess the fundus status and the area of retinal pathologies through the panoramic view and evaluating peripheral retina without requiring extreme rotation of the glob as was generally needed when using prismatic lenses [22]. While working in one membrane, visualization of remote traction with possible advancement of retinal tears or hemorrhage is very important in complex surgeries. Complicated surgeries like dissection of anterior proliferative vitreoretinopathy, air-fluid exchanges, and silicone oil injection both an air-silicone oil exchange and direct PFC-silicone oil exchange can be performed with same system without changing settings.

The WAVs developed in recent years additionally encouraged the utilization of microincisional approaches for plana vitrectomy. Utilizing WAVs, the full-degree dissection of the vitreous base, where remaining vitreous frequently causes failure, can be performed with precise control. The modern WAVs improve the vitreoretinal surgeons' manipulative capacities by giving not just a wide-field perspective of the fundus yet additionally provides good-quality video recording of difficult maneuvers. Sharing these videos in meetings or online platforms with other surgeons helps adding to safety and facilitating the technical troubles.

5. Tamponading agents

Tamponade by medical definition is the utilization of a tampon, which itself is characterized as a plug or tent embedded firmly into a wound to arrest hemorrhage.

With regard to vitreoretinal surgery, tamponade agents are utilized to give surface tension over retinal breaks, which counteracts further liquid stream into the subretinal space until the retinopexy (photocoagulation or cryopexy) gives a lasting chorioretinal attachment. Gases and silicone oils are the most commonly used classes of tamponade agents. Silicone oil was initially used without vitrectomy more as an instrument rather than tamponading agent [23].

In addition to the availability of different viscosities of silicone oil (1000 and 5000 centistokes), heavy silicone oil (Densiron) is also available that sinks in water and hence can be used to tamponade inferior retina [24].

PFC liquids are an important contribution made by Stanley Chang to vitreoretinal surgery [25]. These heavier-than-water liquids are used intraoperatively to facilitate various procedures like inverting the flap of giant retinal tear, performing relaxing retinectomies, displacement of subretinal fluid and blood, floating dislocated intraocular lens, and stabilizing posterior pole for peripheral dissection. PFC liquids are mostly used as intraoperative agents and also sometimes used for long term in spite of its toxicity to retina. Silicone oil is still the best long-term tamponading agent available although the search is going on for a better substitute.

Partially fluorinated alkanes combined with silicone oil and two-staged surgeries that involve removing PFC liquid as a second surgery are discussed in "Surgical techniques" section of this chapter.

6. Intraoperative technologies

6.1 Intraoperative optical coherence tomography

In clinical setting, the noncontact method of cross-sectional imaging of the retina with optical coherence tomography (OCT) became an integral part of evaluation, management, and monitoring of wide range of retinal pathologies since the 2000s. [26]. Development of spectral-domain OCT (SD-OCT) provided improvement in resolution and speed of acquisition, which allowed for more detailed visualization [27]. In addition to its role in clinical management, OCT imaging plays an important role in preoperative surgical planning and postoperative evaluation, especially with epiretinal membranes, macular holes, and rhegmatogenous and tractional retinal detachments. Requirement of upright patient positioning and patient cooperation with the conventional tabletop OCT unit precluded its use in supine patients in the operation room. In 2007 a portable and handheld SD-OCT scanner was developed, which allowed imaging of supine patients. It is mainly used for exams under anesthesia for pediatric patients with various conditions, such as retinopathy of prematurity, albinism, and shaken baby syndrome [28–30].

Development of microscope-mounted OCT devices led to a decrease in image capture time and improvement of reproducibility [31–33]. Although this allowed an easier alignment of the system, but real-time visualization of the tissue and tissue-instrument interactions were not possible until the development of microscope-integrated intraoperative OCT (MiOCT) devices [34, 35]. MiOCT systems incorporate the OCT optical path into the common optical pathway of the surgical microscope, allowing improved targeting and tracking of the scan beam and achieving parfocal and coaxial OCT imaging with the surgical view.

The first publication of MiOCT use in vitreoretinal surgery was in 2010, describing a custom prototype system with a research OCT integrated with a commercially available operating microscope [36]. Several prototypes were developed to be used in clinical vitreoretinal surgery, and some have become commercially available [37, 38]. Currently, three systems are approved by the US Food and Drug

Administration for vitreoretinal surgery in clinical setting (viz., Leica EnFocus, Haag-Streit iOCT, Zeiss RESCAN 700).

Better understanding of the vitreoretinal interface disease and intraoperative changes occurred with different surgical techniques, and tissue manipulation can influence surgical decision-making and possibly lead to improved surgical outcomes. Significant advances in software and hardware of MiOCT systems led to examination of their use for different conditions. In vitreomacular traction repair procedures, MiOCT provides real-time assessment of the strength of vitreomacular adhesions and allows visualization of unroofed cysts, subclinical full-thickness macular hole development, and incomplete peeling of membranes. Intraoperative identification of these subclinical changes may alter the immediate surgical approach, such as prompting the use of gas tamponade and potentially preventing the need for reoperation [39]. In retinal detachment surgery, MiOCT aids in detection of residual subretinal fluid, small retinal breaks, and proliferative vitreoretinopathy membranes and can assist in completion of fluid-air exchange. In tractional retinal detachment surgeries, real-time visualization of the planes may also help achieve more precise delamination and segmentation. MiOCT may also offer benefits to regenerative and gene therapies in the future, improving precision of delivery of a therapeutic agent in subretinal space.

Further software and hardware changes will be necessary to address the current MiOCT systems limitations. Known limitations are related to visualization of OCT data on external screens versus surgical oculars, difficulties with imaging peripheral retina, and light scattering and shadowing from surgical instruments. In systems with inocular heads-up display systems, the size of OCT images and the visual field are limited by the size of the surgical oculars. The use of an external monitor for viewing OCT images provides a larger image, but it requires the surgeon to look away from the surgical field. Additionally, MiOCT systems can cause deterioration of image while evaluating peripheral retina, limiting its use in evaluating peripheral regions. Surgical instruments may lead to light scattering and shadowing, limiting to some degree the real-time visualization of retina manipulation. The amount of shadowing varies depending on instrument material, configuration, thickness, and relative orientation to the optical axis of the OCT [40]. Development of instruments that minimize scatter and shadowing may allow for more precise tissue manipulation. The use of semitransparent rigid plastic material instruments may allow decreased light scatter and improved visibility of adjacent tissue as well as the tissue immediately underlying the instruments [41]. Furthermore, development of new software algorithms may assist in software-based processing of the image to minimize shadowing as well as focusing the OCT image to the area of interest.

6.2 Heads-up surgery

Recent developments in three-dimensional (3D) heads-up vitreoretinal surgery viewing are also gaining popularity. New digitally assisted vitreoretinal surgery systems allow surgeons to maintain a heads-up position instead of having to look down through the microscope oculars. 3D high-dynamic-range cameras mounted in place of the microscope oculars, which are connected to a central processing unit, finally project live feed onto screen.

Reported advantages of this system include high magnification; improved ergonomics for the surgeon; a decrease in required endoillumination through enhanced digital signal processing; improved depth of field; ability to overlay diagnostic studies, including intraoperative OCT data; and enhanced teaching and observation capabilities [42, 43].

Improved ergonomics is the most important advantage of this system. Without the need to lean forward and look into microscope oculars, the surgeon can sit back in the chair and use the backrest for back support. This setup can reduce back and neck strains, especially for long surgeries in complicated cases. Image quality depends on specific conditions, such as distance of the display from the surgeon, angle of the display relative to the surgeon, and minimization of glare. The monitor positioning must be as straight as possible to achieve optimal image quality. Because an assistant sits perpendicular to the patient's head, there is a need for a head turn toward the screen, which may require more time for the assistant to adapt.

With the surgery displayed on the screen, anyone in the room wearing 3D glasses is able to see the details of surgery. This provides an important educational benefit, allowing trainees to observe exactly what the surgeon is doing.

One of the important benefits of digital image processing is being able to use lower endoillumination levels by increasing the camera aperture settings, potentially decreasing phototoxicity, especially for macular cases. Another benefit includes real-time image processing and color manipulation, which can allow better visualization of the vitreous and decreased glare. The increase in depth of field and wider field of view also helps in complex cases, such as proliferative vitreoretinopathy involved in complex retinal detachment, intraocular foreign body, and scleral-fixated intraocular lens cases. Further developments in real-time digital signal processing area also could enhance this technology more.

In summary, new developments in MiOCT systems offer immediate imageguidance for vitreoretinal surgeons; they may improve our understanding of effects of surgical manipulation on tissues and possibly allow us to explain and predict variations in postoperative visual outcomes. Heads-up digitally assisted surgical viewing systems change the ergonomics as well as enhance the viewing and teaching capabilities in the operating rooms.

7. Dyes

For vitreoretinal surgery, vital dyes enable easier identification of the semitransparent preretinal membranes. Current recommendations for the application of dyes during vitreoretinal surgery indicate that indocyanine green, infracyanine green, brilliant blue, and bromophenol blue may be the best stains for the internal limiting membrane (ILM), while trypan blue may be preferred for staining the glial tissues like epiretinal membrane [44].

In regard to the toxicity issues in chromovitrectomy, a large number of experimental and clinical investigations in this challenging field with vital dyes have yielded some controversial results, but preliminary conclusions may be drawn at this time. Indocyanine green has been proven to be toxic to the retina, and brilliant blue showed a better safety profile and could protect against apoptosis, at least in vitro [44, 45].

Each vital dye injected intravitreally poses a rather dose-dependent toxicity to the retinal tissue. Furthermore, there is solid proof that light exposure, osmolarity, and existence of ions, for example, Na + and iodine, may apply further harm to the retina. Along these lines, general proposals for all vital dyes incorporate injection of a very low amount onto the retina, staying away from long macular exposure to endoillumination and expulsion of sodium and iodine from dye solutions.

8. Endoscopic vitrectomy

Endoscopic vitrectomy provides direct visualization of the posterior segment with a directional camera, allowing surgeons to bypass compromised anterior segments, opacified corneas, and media opacities. Additionally, the ability to direct the visualization from the pars plana allows surgeons a method to visualize the anterior retina, ciliary body, and posterior iris surface in their natural anatomic configuration. New techniques are continually being described that demonstrate how endoscopic vitrectomy is beneficial to the retinal surgeon. The most obvious advantage of endoscopic vitrectomy is the ability to provide excellent visualization in eyes with the opacified cornea and lens. It may also allow extreme peripheral panretinal photocoagulation in the patients with peripheral ischemic retinopathies. It allows endoscopic cyclophotocoagulation in patients with glaucoma, either at the time of cataract surgery or as a stand-alone procedure [46].

There are limitations to utilization of an endoscope, such as limited field of view, which requires some adjustment given the familiarity with wide-field viewing systems. Additionally, the view is monocular, so the surgeon must utilize other cues, such as focus, size, and light intensity, to compensate [47]. The free rotation ability of the endoscope probe creates difficulty with orientation, making movements within the eye challenging, especially in the learning period of surgeon. Despite these limitations, endoscopic vitrectomy is a useful addition to the retinal surgeon's armamentarium. The ability to bypass media opacities and to visualize structures otherwise not visible creates opportunities for unique surgical interventions in complicated and even inoperable surgical situations.

9. Surgical techniques

9.1 Scleral buckle

There are variable techniques used for vitreoretinal surgeries, and they are all being continuously refined. Scleral buckle is an example originated in the 1950s but is still developing. Some modifications are still being reported on scleral buckle; as mentioned earlier in this chapter, using chandelier lightning and WAV systems, instead of indirect ophthalmoscopy, becomes the preferred method of choice in many retina clinics. Chandelier assistance obviates the need for indirect ophthalmoscopy and capitalizes on the advantages provided by the operating microscope and modern wide-angle viewing systems such as an improved view of the peripheral retina with oblique lighting to perhaps improve identification of peripheral breaks. Wide-field viewing may also make subretinal fluid needle drainage safer as it may decrease the risk of losing the view of the needle, which may occur with indirect ophthalmoscopy. Moreover, chandelier buckling allows trainers to view same with the surgeon and is better for teaching purposes. In addition, chandelier-assisted scleral buckling permits standard microscope-facilitated recording of the important surgical steps of this procedure, which also facilitates dissemination of scleral buckling techniques. Many authors of the published literature regarding this technique also mention the improved ergonomics of using the operating microscope to perform examination and treatment of retinal breaks instead of indirect ophthalmoscopy [13].

Classic scleral buckle surgery normally incorporates a substantial or 360-degree peritomy. A recent report detailed a method for segmental buckle through a small conjunctival opening, which was utilized in uncomplicated rhegmatogenous retinal detachments [48]. This surgical technique incorporates performing 5 to 6 mm radial conjunctival cut in close to the retinal break without cutting the limbal conjunctiva and Tenon's layer, followed by cryopexy and implantation of a small segmental buckle that was sutured through the conjunctival opening. Cosmetic and functional results were reported as quick and superb.

9.2 Suprachoroidal buckle

Another imaginative method has been depicted for suprachoroidal buckle surgery. In this method, a lighted catheter is inserted into the suprachoroidal space and placed to any desired area over the breaks; there, an enduring hyaluronic acid filler can be injected to create choroidal indentation. This can be performed with or without pars plana vitrectomy and has been reported effective for the treatment of patients with retinal detachment [49, 50].

9.3 Macular surgeries

Inverted internal limiting membrane (ILM) flap technique has been reported to improve the closure rates of large and persistent macular holes [51]. This technique has recently been suggested for the treatment of macular retinal detachment due to macular holes in highly myopic eyes in which macular holes are relatively difficult to close [52]. Higher rates of macular hole closure and retinal attachment, and additionally a little yet noteworthy improvement in visual acuity, were accomplished with this procedure [53]. It has been recommended that the inverted ILM flap stimulates the multiplication of glial cells that helps in closing the macular hole.

Another interesting new technique has been reported for the treatment of macular folds. Detachment of macula performed by subretinal injection of balanced salt solution and minimal amount of filtered air. Under these conditions, the action of gravity of the PFC liquid and with an active globe rotation has been reported to achieve successful flattening of the macula [54].

9.4 Pars plana vitrectomy for retinal detachment

Development of improved retinopexy methods which could produce immediate chorioretinal adhesion of sufficient strength may obviate the need for long-term tamponade. Recent studies have evaluated the potential of high-frequency electric welding was able to create an immediate retinopexy equal in strength to mature laser retinopexy, which takes about 2 weeks to achieve maximum adhesion [55]. Previously reported methods to achieve adhesion include the development of biocompatible glues, analogous to fibrin [56, 57]. The elimination of long-term gas tamponade and elimination of the need for patient positioning may be the next major advance in retinal detachment surgery.

An interesting technique has been suggested to prevent passage of PFC liquid into the subretinal space. After performing vitrectomy, viscoelastic material was injected over areas where confluent retinal folds were formed with possible retinal breaks. This protective layer still prevents PFC liquid from entering the subretinal space [58].

Pneumatic retinopexy is also an option for retinal detachments caused by within one-clock hour of the retinal arc in the upper two-thirds of the retina and sufficiently clears media to rule out the presence of other retinal breaks. In cases when cryopexy is not performed, it may be difficult to visualize and localize the retinal breaks after the intravitreal gas injection. A recent report of preoperative laser marking of the ora serrata at the meridians of the break made it easy to find after pneumatic retinopexy has been performed [59]. The gas used for pneumatic retinopexy is usually C3F8 or SF6 at 100% expansile concentration, which allows for injection of a relatively small volume of gas that later expands and can cover a greater area of the retinal surface [60]. The advantage of using air is its faster rate of elimination, which allows the patients to regain good visual acuity sooner (5 days versus 2–4 weeks with the gases).

A recent study reported on proliferative vitreoretinopathy retinal detachment cases, intravitreal conbercept administrated a week prior to surgery. Administration of conbercept, a recombinant fusion protein with antivascular endothelial growth factor (VEGF) activity, was found to reduce the rate of intraoperative bleeding, which can facilitate the management of these difficult cases.

Partially fluorinated alkanes that were introduced as long-term heavy tamponades, which are heavier than water, may be of benefit especially in the treatment of inferior retinal detachment cases. One of these is F6H8, which is not routinely used due to its early dispersion and emulsification with consequent inflammatory response. A study investigated its use in combination with silicone oil, in a series of eyes with inferior retinal detachment, where F6H8 was used to flatten the retina and was later partially mixed with silicone oil for long-term tamponade. This combination resulted in a clear tamponade allowing postoperative visualization of the retina, with no emulsification, inflammation, or other complications [61].

Another option is planning a stage two procedure; after the initial vitrectomy was performed, PFC liquid is infused overlying the optic nerve head until a complete fill of the vitreous cavity was achieved. Patients were instructed to avoid facedown positioning. The staged second procedure was performed 16 to 21 days after all laser scars were noted to be pigmented, with a silicone soft-tip extrusion cannula to remove PFC liquid. Repeated fluid-air/air-fluid exchange was used to remove all PFC from the vitreous cavity. When present anterior chamber PFC also has to be removed [62].

10. Conclusion

The new developments in surgical instruments, machines, trocars, viewing systems, and surgical techniques played significant role in decreasing complications and improving outcomes of modern vitreoretinal surgeries. There are still some problems to solve in modern vitreoretinal surgeries, like finding a better tamponade that does not have necessity to remove from the eye yet also stabilize the retinal breaks better with good visual recovery from the first postoperative day. Also better drugs needed to be discovered to prevent proliferative vitreoretinopathy and hypotony. In addition there are new achievements in stem cell therapies and artificial retinal implants. The progress in vitreoretinal surgery area is ongoing faster than ever before. In the near future, surgery will be an option for a variety of different vitreoretinal pathologies, including cases we classify as inoperable today.

Conflict of interest

The author did not have a conflict of interest for any products mentioned in the above text.

DOI: http://dx.doi.org/10.5772/intechopen.83019

Author details

Baris Komur
Istanbul Haseki Education and Research Hospital, Turkey

*Address all correspondence to: bkomur@gmail.com

References

[1] Machemer R, Norton E. Vitrectomy, a pars plana approach II. Clinical experience. Modern Problems in Ophthalmology. 1972;**10**:178-185

[2] Charles S. The history of vitrectomy: Innovation and evolution. Retina Today. 2008;**4**:27-29

[3] Charles S. Endophotocoagulation. Retina. 1981;**1**:117-120

[4] Mitsui K, Kogo J, Takeda H, Shiono A, Sasaki H, Munemasa Y, et al. Comparative study of 27-gauge vs. 25-gauge vitrectomy for epiretinal membrane. Eye. 2016;**30**:538-544

[5] Chaves de Oliveira PR, Berger AR, Chow DR. Vitreoretinal instruments: Vitrectomy cutters, endoillumination and wide-angle viewing systems. International Journal of Retina and Vitreous. 2016;**2**:28

[6] Mariotti C, Nicolai M, Saitta A, Orsini E, Viti F, Skrami E, et al. Standard cut rate 25-gauge vitrectomy versus ultrahigh-speed 25-gauge system in core vitrectomy: A randomized clinical trial. Retina. 2016;**36**:127104

[7] Pavlidis M. Two-dimensional cutting (TDC) vitrectome: In vivo flow assessment and prospective clinical study evaluating core vitrectomy efficiency versus standard vitrectome. Journal of Ophthalmology. 2016;**2016**:3849316

[8] Pastor S, Bonshek R, Luciane I, Zambrano I, Carlin P, Stanga PE. New prototype of ultrasound harmonics vitrector (UHV) histopathological findings: First report. Investigative Ophthalmology and Visual Science. 2015;**56**:394

[9] Stanga PE, Pastor S, Zambrano I, Carlin P. New prototype of ultrasound harmonics vitrector (UHV) fluidics analysis: First report. Investigative Ophthalmology and Visual Science. 2015;**56**:385

[10] Sakaguchi H, Oshima Y. Considering the illumination choices in vitreoretinal surgery. Retinal Physician. 2012;**9**:26-31

[11] Chow DR. The evolution of endoillumination. Developments in Ophthalmology. 2014;**54**:77-86

[12] Aydin B, Dinç E, Yilmaz SN, Altiparmak UE, Yülek F, Ertekin S, et al. Retinal endoilluminator toxicity of xenon and light-emitting diode (LED) light source: Rabbit model. Cutaneous and Ocular Toxicology. 2014;**33**:192-196

[13] Seider MI, Nomides RE, Hahn P, Mruthyunjaya P, Mahmoud TH. Scleral buckling with chandelier illumination. Journal of Ophthalmic & Vision Research. 2016;**11**:304-309

[14] Bilgin S, Kayikcioglu O. Chandelier retroillumination-assisted cataract surgery during vitrectomy. Eye (London). 2016;**30**:1123-1125

[15] Chang S. Transitioning to microincisional vitrectomy surgery. Retina Today. 2008;**4**:5-6

[16] De Juan E Jr, Hickingbotham D. Refinements in microinstrumentation for vitreous surgery. American Journal of Ophthalmology. 1990;**109**:218-220

[17] Fujii GY, De Juan E Jr, Humayun MS, Pieramici DJ, Chang TS, Awh C, et al. A new 25-gauge instrument system for transconjunctival sutureless vitrectomy surgery. Ophthalmology. 2002;**109**:1807-1812

[18] Abulon D, Charles M. The impact of valved and non-valved cannula on intraoperative fluid dynamics and vitreous. In: 14th Euretina Congress; September 11-14. London; 2014

[19] Spitznas M. A binocular indirect ophthalmomicroscope (BIOM) for non-contact wide-angle vitreous surgery. Graefe's Archive for Clinical and Experimental Ophthalmology. 1987;**225**:13-15

[20] Peyman GA. A new wide-angle irrigating contact lens for pars plana vitrectomy. Canadian Journal of Ophthalmology. 1988;**23**:150-155

[21] Kadonosono K. Achieving wide angle view during vitrectomy. Retina Today. 2011;**6**:43-45

[22] Chalam KV, Shah VA. Optics of wide-angle panoramic viewing system-assisted vitreous surgery. Survey of Ophthalmology. 2004;**49**:437-445

[23] Cibis PA. Treatment of retinal detachment by injection of silicon oil into the vitreous body. Ber Zusammenkunft Dtsch Ophthalmol Ges. 1965;**66**:433-434

[24] Stappler T, Heinmann H, Gibran SK, Groenewald C, Pearce IA, Wong D. Densiron-68 heavy silicone oil in cases of PVR. Anatomical and functional outcomes. Der Ophthalmologe. 2009;**106**:320-326

[25] Coll GE, Chang S, Sun J, Wieland MR, Berrocal MH. Perfluorocarbon liquid in the management of retinal detachment with proliferative vitreoretinopathy. Ophthalmology. 1995;**102**:630-638

[26] Huang D, Swanson EA, Lin CP, Schuman JS, Stinson WG, Chang W, et al. Optical coherence tomography. Science. 1991;**254**:1178-1181

[27] Gabriele ML, Wollstein G, Ishikawa H, Xu J, Kim J, Kagemann L, et al. Three dimensional optical coherence tomography imaging: Advantages and advances. Progress in Retinal and Eye Research. 2010;**29**:556-579

[28] Muni RH, Kohly RP, Sohn EH, Lee TC. Hand-held spectral domain optical coherence tomography finding in shaken-baby syndrome. Retina. 2010;**30**:45-50

[29] Chong GT, Farsiu S, Freedman SF, Sarin N, Koreishi AF, Izatt JA. et al. Abnormal foveal morphology in ocular albinism imaged with spectral-domain optical coherence tomography. Archives of Ophthalmology. 2009;**127**:37-44

[30] Muni RH, Kohly RP, Charonis AC, Lee TC. Retinoschisis detected with handheld spectral-domain optical coherence tomography in neonates with advanced retinopathy of prematurity. Archives of Ophthalmology. 2010;**128**:57-62

[31] Ray R, Barañano DE, Fortun JA, Schwent BJ, Cribbs BE, Bergstrom CS, et al. Intraoperative microscope-mounted spectral domain optical coherence tomography for evaluation of retinal anatomy during macular surgery. Ophthalmology. 2011;**118**:2212-2217

[32] Binder S, Falkner-Radler CI, Hauger C, Matz H, Glittenberg C. Feasibility of intrasurgical spectral-domain optical coherence tomography. Retina. 2011;**31**:1332-1336

[33] Ehlers JP, Tao YK, Farsiu S, Maldonado R, Izatt JA, Toth CA. Visualization of real-time intraoperative maneuvers with a microscope-mounted spectral domain optical coherence tomography system. Retina. 2013;**33**:232-236

[34] Hahn P, Carrasco-Zevallos O, Cunefare D, Migacz J, Farsiu S, Izatt JA, et al. Intrasurgical human retinal imaging with manual instrument tracking using a microscope-integrated spectral-domain optical coherence tomography device. Translational Vision Science & Technology. 2015;**4**:1

[35] Hahn P, Migacz J, O'Connell R, Izatt JA, Toth CA. Unprocessed real-time imaging of vitreoretinal surgical maneuvers using a microscope-integrated spectral-domain optical coherence tomography system. Graefe's Archive for Clinical and Experimental Ophthalmology. 2013;**251**:213-220

[36] Tao YK, Ehlers JP, Toth CA, Izatt JA. Intraoperative spectral domain optical coherence tomography for vitreoretinal surgery. Optics Letters. 2010;**35**:3315-3317

[37] Runkle A, Srivastava SK, Ehlers JP. Microscope-integrated OCT feasibility and utility with the EnFocus system in the DISCOVER study. Ophthalmic Surgery, Lasers and Imaging Retina. 2017;**48**:216-222

[38] Hahn P, Migacz J, O'Donnell R, Day S, Lee A, Lin P, et al. Preclinical evaluation and intraoperative human retinal imaging with a high-resolution microscope-integrated spectral domain optical coherence tomography device. Retina. 2013;**33**:1328-1337

[39] Ehlers JP, Tam T, Kaiser PK, Martin DF, Smith GM, Srivastava SK. Utility of intraoperative optical coherence tomography during vitrectomy surgery for vitreomacular traction syndrome. Retina. 2014;**34**:1341-1346

[40] Ehlers JP, Ohr MP, Kaiser PK, Srivastava SK. Novel microarchitectural dynamics in rhegmatogenous retinal detachments identified with intraoperative optical coherence tomography. Retina. 2013;**33**:1428-1434

[41] Ehlers JP, Uchida A, Srivastava SK. Intraoperative optical coherence tomography-compatible surgical instruments for real-time image-guided ophthalmic surgery. The British Journal of Ophthalmology. 2017;**101**:1306-1308

[42] Eckardt C, Paulo EB. Heads-up surgery for vitreoretinal procedures: An experimental and clinical study. Retina. 2016;**36**:137-147

[43] Skinner CS, Riemann CD. "Heads up" digitally assisted surgical viewing for retinal detachment repair in a patient with severe kyphosis. Retinal Cases and Brief Reports. 2018;**12**:257-259

[44] Penha FM, Pons M, Costa EF, Barros NM, Rodrigues EB, Cardoso EB, et al. Retinal pigmented epithelial cells cytotoxicity and apoptosis through activation of the mitochondrial intrinsic pathway: Role of indocyanine green, brilliant blue and implications for chromovitrectomy. PLoS One. 2013;**8**:e64094

[45] Penha FM, Pons M, Costa Ede P, Rodrigues EB, Maia M, Marin-Castaño ME, et al. Effect of vital dyes on retinal pigmented epithelial cell viability and apoptosis: Implications for chromovitrectomy. Ophthalmologica. 2013;**230**:41-50

[46] Marra KV, Yonekawa Y, Papakostas TD. Indications and techniques of endoscope assisted vitrectomy. Journal of Ophthalmic & Vision Research. 2013;**8**:282-290

[47] Lee GD, Goldberg RA, Heier JS. Endoscopy-assisted vitrectomy and membrane dissection of anterior proliferative vitreoretinopathy for chronic hypotony after previous retinal detachment repair. Retina. 2016;**36**:1058-1063

[48] Jin H, Zhang Q , Zhao P. Minimal in situ conjunctival incision for segmental scleral buckling surgery. Ophthalmic Surgery, Lasers and Imaging Retina. 2014;**45**:574-576

[49] El Rayes EN, Oshima Y. Suprachoroidal buckling for retinal detachment. Retina. 2013;**33**:1073-1075

[50] El Rayes EN, Mikhail M, El Cheweiky H, Elsawah K, Maia A.

Suprachoroidal buckling for the management of rhegmatogenous retinal detachments secondary to peripheral retinal breaks. Retina. 2016;**4**:622-629

[51] Michalewska Z, Michalewski J, Adelman RA, Nawrocki J. Inverted internal limiting membrane flap technique for large macular holes. Ophthalmology. 2010;**117**:2018-2025

[52] Okuda T, Higashide T, Kobayashi K, Ikuno Y, Sugiyama K. Macular hole closure over residual subretinal fluid by an inverted internal limiting membrane flap technique in patients with macular hole retinal detachment in high myopia. Retinal Cases and Brief Reports. 2016;**10**:140-144

[53] Matsumura T, Takamura Y, Tomomatsu T, Arimura S, Gozawa M, Kobori A, et al. Comparison of the inverted internal limiting membrane flap technique and the internal limiting membrane peeling for macular hole with retinal detachment. PLoS One. 2016;**11**:e0165068

[54] Barale PO, Mora P, Errera MH, Ores R, Pâques M, Sahel JA. Treatment of macular folds complicating retinal detachment surgery using air for retinal unfolding. Retinal Cases and Brief Reports. 2018;**12**:228-230

[55] Umanets N, Pasyechnikova NV, Naumenko VA, Henrich PB. High-frequency electric welding: A novel method for improved immediate chorioretinal adhesion in vitreoretinal surgery. Graefe's Archive for Clinical and Experimental Ophthalmology. 2014;**252**: 1697-1703

[56] Chen T, Janjua R, McDermott MK, Bernstein SL, Steidl SM, Payne GF. Gelatin-based biomimetic tissue adhesive. Potential for retinal reattachment. Journal of Biomedical Materials Research Part B: Applied Biomaterials. 2006;**77**:416-422

[57] Margalit E, Fujii GY, Lai JC, Gupta P, Chen SJ, Shyu JS, et al. Bioadhesives for intraocular use. Retina. 2000;**20**(5):469-477

[58] Yamakiri K, Uchino E, Sakamoto T. Soft shell technique during vitrectomy for proliferative vitreoretinopathy. Graefe's Archive for Clinical and Experimental Ophthalmology. 2016;**254**(6):1069-1073

[59] Yan P, Minaker S, Mandelcorn ED. Laser marking of the meridian of retinal breaks at the ora: A novel technique for pneumatic retinopexy. Ophthalmic Surgery, Lasers and Imaging Retina. 2016;**47**:570-572

[60] Yee KM, Sebag J. Long-term results of office-based pneumatic retinopexy using pure air. British Journal of Ophthalmology. 2011;**95**:1728-1730

[61] Tosi GM, Marigliani D, Bacci T, Romeo N, Balestrazzi A, Martone G, et al. F6H8 as an intraoperative tool and F6H8/silicone oil as a postoperative tamponade in inferior retinal detachment with inferior PVR. Journal of Ophthalmology. 2014;**2014**:956831

[62] Sigler EJ, Randolph JC, Calzada JI, Charles S. Pars plana vitrectomy with medium-term postoperative perfluoro-N-octane for recurrent inferior retinal detachment complicated by advanced proliferative vitreoretinopathy. Retina. 2013;**33**:791-797